BEHIND THE DOOR OF DELUSION

BEHIND THE DOOR OF DELUSION

BY "INMATE WARD 8"

Edited, With an
Introduction and Afterword by

WILLIAM W. SAVAGE, JR. AND
JAMES H. LAZALIER

UNIVERSITY PRESS OF COLORADO

Copyright © 1994 by the University Press of Colorado
Copyright © 1932 by the Macmillan Company

Published by the University Press of Colorado
P.O. Box 849
Niwot, Colorado 80544

The University Press of Colorado is a cooperative publishing enterprise supported, in part, by Adams State College, Colorado State University, Fort Lewis College, Mesa State College, Metropolitan State College of Denver, University of Colorado, University of Northern Colorado, University of Southern Colorado, and Western State College of Colorado.

Library of Congress Cataloging-in-Publication Data

Woodson, Marle, 1882-1933.
    Behind the door of delusion / by Inmate Ward 8 ; introduction and afterword by William W. Savage and James H. Lazalier.
      p. cm.
    Originally published: New York : Macmillan, 1932.
    ISBN 0-87081-314-5 (cloth).—ISBN 0-87081-315-3 (paper)
    1. Psychiatric hospitals—Sociological aspects—Case studies.
2. Psychiatric hospital patients—Case studies. 3. Psychiatric hospital care—Case studies. I. Title.
RC439.W65   1994
362.2'1—dc20
[B]
                                                                                              94-8412
                                                                                                CIP

The paper used in this publication meets the minimum requirements of the American National Standard for Information Sciences—Permanence of Paper for Printed Library Materials. ANSI Z39.48–1984
∞

10 9 8 7 6 5 4 3 2 1

*Dedicated to a better understanding
of those on the inside by those
who are not yet locked in.*

Contents

	Introduction	ix
	Introduction to the Original	1
	Prologue	3
I	Checked In	7
II	The Lonely Drag	14
III	Our Sane Insane	24
IV	Lights and Shadows	35
V	Flying Feet	45
VI	Bars and Strong Arms	54
VII	Unrestrained Senses	62
VIII	Insidious Fears	69
IX	Pot Pourri	77
X	Sleeping Sickness	89
XI	Introspection	100
XII	The Halting Advance	107
XIII	Silhouettes	118
XIV	The Sterilization Spectre	125
XV	In Self Defense	136
XVI	Futile	144
XVII	Jam on the Brakes	150
XVIII	Debts of Others	155
XIX	Dress Parade	159
XX	Hung on the Line	165
XXI	Spin of the Wheel	171
	Afterword	176

INTRODUCTION

WILLIAM W. SAVAGE, JR. AND JAMES H. LAZALIER

Behind the Door of Delusion is the memoir of a journalist whose friends committed him to an Oklahoma mental hospital in the early 1930s in a final, desperate effort to rid him of the craving for alcohol that had been his recurring problem and was, as he entered the sixth decade of his life, quite obviously about to kill him. It is a powerful book, an uncommon social document of Depression-era America that provides insight into political and economic forces affecting the maintenance of a neglected underclass. And it suggests that long before the Joads of John Steinbeck's imagination made their pilgrimage to California, other Okies had fled hard times on a narrower road—one that led, not west, but deep inside themselves.

When Macmillan published *Behind the Door of Delusion* in 1932, its title page attributed the work only to "Inmate Ward 8," posing a mystery of minuscule proportions to eastern reviewers who cared nothing about the author and wished merely to exercise themselves by attacking or defending modern psychiatric practices.[1] West of the Mississippi, especially in the vicinity of Oklahoma, the identity of "Inmate Ward 8" was better known, inasmuch as the journalists who reviewed the book could certainly recognize one of their own. They knew the author to be Marle Woodson, one-time foreign correspondent for Associated Press and lately a writer for the *Tulsa World*.[2]

Born Marion Marle in 1879 to an affluent family (his father was a lawyer who would become a judge, his mother a Southern belle), Woodson spent some of his formative years in Oklahoma Territory.[3] Around the turn of the century he enrolled in Oklahoma A & M College (now Oklahoma State University), informing what acquaintances later called a brilliant mind, but participating as well in track, wrestling, and football. After graduation, he played minor-league baseball for several years, perhaps to finance a bit of postgraduate study.

In 1908, at age twenty-nine, Woodson became president of Connell State School of Agriculture, at Helena, Oklahoma, in Alfalfa County, not far from the Kansas line. He was the youngest college president in Oklahoma, friends boasted; but it was not a distinction that would excuse him from dealing with the institution's profound fiscal problems. (Within a decade, Connell would close its doors permanently, in consequence of a budget-minded governor's refusal to sanction further appropriations for it). Brief administrative experience was enough—if not too much—for Woodson, and by 1912, as proof that he was sufficiently talented to do whatever he pleased, he was reporting from the Balkans and India in what would become a five-year stint with Associated Press. Thereafter, he returned to Oklahoma and a job writing for the *Tulsa Tribune*.

Biographical material on Marle Woodson is scarce, and what exists seems awfully threadbare. Evidently he changed jobs often during the next several years, perhaps owing to bouts with alcoholism. At one point, he worked for a newspaper in Pasadena, California, becoming so enamored of the city's annual celebration of the rose that he later sought to re-create it in Oklahoma. He organized and for several years managed the Tulsa Rose Carnival, acquiring in the process the status of civic leader and making the acquaintance of virtually every mover and shaker in northeastern Oklahoma.[4] In the late 1920s he was by most accounts certainly a prominent citizen, albeit one who admitted to staying up nights and imbibing vast quantities of liquor at parties of one kind or another, or by himself if it came to that. We know from his comments in *Behind the Door of Delusion* that over the years he spent thousands of dollars for repeated stays in any number of private hospitals and sanitariums, all in the vain attempt to achieve and maintain sobriety.

There was hideous irony in Woodson's situation. Prohibition, included in an early amendment to the state constitution, had been the ostensible rule in Oklahoma since 1907, some thirteen years before the Volstead Act and the Eighteenth Amendment sought to muffle the anticipated roaring of the twenties. But neither federal nor state laws presented any obstacle to the thirsty Woodson or anybody else with a few dollars and a bootlegger's address, especially in Tulsa. The city was periodically awash in enough oil money to keep the night-life going, even through the downside of eastern Oklahoma's boom-and-bust economy; and ever since statehood Tulsa had been the proverbial wide-open town. The Eighteenth Amendment made no difference one way or the other. Local officials simply had no interest in enforcing liquor laws, and there were never enough federal agents around to do the job.[5] Marle Woodson could drink to excess in a bone-dry state, unmolested except perhaps by his conscience and a few of his friends.

Those friends prevailed at last in 1931, when Woodson, then aged 52, seemed particularly bent on drinking himself into the grave.[6] He was in no condition to protest when they took him before a sympathetic judge who agreed that the journalist be committed to Eastern Oklahoma Hospital at Vinita, about sixty miles northeast of Tulsa. The idea was to put him somewhere arid and keep him there long enough to overcome his thirst.

Prohibition, nowhere else effective in Oklahoma, might work within the walls of a mental hospital.

The judge who committed him understood that Woodson was not insane, according to the criteria established for institution-alization; nor was he mentally defective or epileptic. The staff at Vinita understood it as well. And Woodson, for his part, came to know that he was hardly unique but merely another of the many "sane insane" who populated what he preferred to call an asylum. Later, some reviewers of his book would complain about the hypocrisy of locking a drunk in a mental hospital on the pretext that he was crazy; but nobody pointed to the hypocrisy of Prohibition.[7]

Among the several things that caught Woodson's attention and thus found mention in his story was the rather dramatic recent increase in the number of patients housed at the Vinita facility. The Depression seemed to be at the bottom of things—and to understand Woodson's context it is well to remember that Oklahoma had experienced a decade of depression in agriculture before the Wall Street calamity of October 1929 ushered in the "Great Depression" that named the thirties. True, there were inmates who had once been the custodians of fortunes, and losing their minds had been a consequence of losing their money. But more common were the people, old and infirm, perhaps, or young and simpleminded, whose families simply could no longer afford to care for them. In the sad and sorry world of rural hard times, one who could not work and contribute something to the family's income was one who could not be allowed to eat. Our images of the Great Depression, whether of somber men in breadlines or soup kitchens, or of Busby Berkeley's platinum chorines singing "We're in the Money," must now include the ones conveyed by Woodson of the blameless unproductive whose handicap is not their unemployment but their unemployability. They were turned over to the state in the faint hope (but even so, a better one than families might otherwise have had) that the state could sustain them.

When Marle Woodson entered Eastern Oklahoma Hospital, the inmate population numbered 1,672, or almost 15 percent above capacity.[8] Oklahoma spent an average of $19.32 per month on each patient at Vinita during 1930, approximately one-third of that amount contributing to staff salaries and two-thirds going to maintain the inmates. Of the $12.60-per-patient monthly maintenance, $7.05 was spent for food, even though the hospital operated its own farm and produced most of the eggs, beef, pork, milk, and vegetables the patients consumed. Assuming that hospital budgets mirrored even dimly the real world, we understand at once that about $85 made the difference between keeping relatives at home or committing them to a mental institution. The hospitals provided a "safety net" for the impoverished well in advance of the better-advertised ones to be generated by Franklin Roosevelt's New Deal. As places of sanctuary and safe harbor for the dispossessed, they perhaps deserved Woodson's label of "asylum." It is not inappropriate to recall Steinbeck's Tom Joad enumerating the advantages of life in the penitentiary over life on the family farm: Prison offered regular meals and electricity and indoor plumbing, whereas home had no such amenities. Surely the mental institutions deserved similar endorsement on those counts.

Withal, Eastern Oklahoma Hospital was still a facility for the mentally ill—and, as Woodson indicated, the sexually diseased—and inmates were there to be segregated from the world of "normal" folk, and, if it were possible, to be cured. Established by politicians and run by clinicians, it could never escape political consideration. Woodson's discussion of the state's 1931 sterilization law (see Chapter XIV) limns the political context of inmate existence. The legislative view was that, if the doctors decided it was best for the patient and for society, any male patient under the age of sixty-five and any female patient under the age of forty-seven could be sterilized prior to discharge, thus eliminating from future generations such things as congenital idiocy. The irony, of course, was that an inmate could leave the hospital in only two ways: sane, or in a casket. To be discharged, one must first be cured of his or her illness; but even so, sterilization might be ordered. A "cured" person who refused sterilization could not be discharged. Woodson's picture of supposed crazy people disputing among themselves the law's double-bind is poignant indeed.

Woodson began writing his book as soon as he emerged from the initial stages of alcohol withdrawal. Detoxification brought him an eloquence and felicity of style unanticipated by his most recent journalism.[9] Whether sobriety or inspiration made it so, *Behind the Door of Delusion* would become Marle Woodson's masterpiece. Woodson advertised it to Macmillan as containing "plenty of pathos . . . glimpses behind the curtains of obsession-torn minds, the undying hope, close hugged, and never relinquished, of 'going home.'"[10] Though the editors at Macmillan were sufficiently impressed to request the manuscript, nothing in Woodson's letter of inquiry could have prepared them for his portraits of Whizbang Mabel, the Amazon who invented original vulgarities whenever she spoke; of Blondy, the demented man who kept trying to escape through he kitchen door; of the Concrete Man and the Spider, who thought that was what they were; of Talking Louis, issuing instructions to the British royal family through an imaginary young woman; or of the beknighted patient who played both parts in a prizefight and ended each performance by knocking himself out. It was pathos that might have been fiction, except for Woodson's assurances to the editors that it was "the kind that really exists."

Behind the Door of Delusion is strong stuff. Few who read it will be unmoved by the story of Joe and his mother in the chapter entitled

"Futile," or by Woodson's own account of his life with Constance, the frivolous party girl who would not abandon him. For all its merit as a social document, its value as history or as literature, the book is almost unbearably sad. Readers are forewarned. There is no happy ending. There is no satisfaction to be derived from Woodson's speculation about the future with Constance. Indeed, the book mirrors tragedy in more ways than one; but let us pause now to read what Woodson wrote, and let us plan to meet again in the Afterword.

NOTES

We express appreciation to Sharon Saulmon of the Learning Resources Center at Rose State College and to Shirley Gidley of the Tulsa City-County Library Periodicals Department for their assistance in obtaining reference material; to Frank Parman of Norman, Oklahoma, who knows more than anybody about his state's literary history; and to Glenda Madden and Kimberly Wiar, also of Norman, for finding Marle Woodson a better home.

1. See, for example, John Rathbone Oliver, "The Abnormal in Fact and Fiction," *The Saturday Review of Literature* (November 26, 1932), p. 272.

2. See Joseph A. Brandt's review in *The Sooner Magazine* (October 1932), pp. 30–32.

3. Biographical material herein has been pieced together from Mary Hays Marable and Elaine Boylan, *A Handbook of Oklahoma Writers* (Norman: University of Oklahoma Press, 1939), pp. 213–16, various reviews of *Behind the Door of Delusion*, and Woodson's obituary notices.

4. Marle Woodson, "Tulsa's Rose Carnival," *My Oklahoma* (May 1927), p. 43.

5. See the discussion in Jimmie Lewis Franklin, *Born Sober: Prohibition in Oklahoma, 1907–1959* (Norman: University of Oklahoma Press, 1971), especially Chapters V–VI.

6. Marable and Boylan, p. 213, give the date as 1930, but Woodson's Associated Press obituary set the date at 1931. In Woodson's book, he spoke of leaving Eastern at the end of a year; the book itself was published in the fall of 1932; and we know that Woodson was still working for the *Tulsa World* in January 1931. Had Woodson been committed and released before that date, there would seem to have been little point in maintaining his anonymity as "Inmate Ward 8" almost two years later. It seems clear that Woodson submitted his manuscript to Macmillan while he was

still a patient at Eastern, and we have reconstructed the chronology with that in mind.

7. Oliver, "The Abnormal in Fact and Fiction." Robert Morss Lovett, "That Way Lies Madness," *The New Republic* (September 21, 1932), p. 159, represented those reviewers who seemingly had no opinion but believed that the book was surely an exposé of something, even if they were not certain what it was. In Lovett's case Woodson received faint praise for not exaggerating about the insane as novelists and reformers generally did.

8. Information about Eastern Oklahoma Hospital here and hereinafter is taken from statistics in *State Mental Hospitals in Oklahoma: A Preliminary Study of Present Facilities and Conditions* (Oklahoma City: Oklahoma Planning and Resources Board, Division of State Planning, 1937).

9. See, for example, Marle Woodson, "The Creek Stomp Dance," *Tulsa Daily World*, January 15, 1928, p. 6; "Tulsan Owns Vast Cattle Ranch in the 'Vanishing West,'" *Tulsa Daily World*, September 15, 1929, p. 7; and "Sam Brown—Last of the Euchee Guardsmen," *Tulsa Daily World*, February 1, 1931, magazine section.

10. The letter is reproduced in Marable and Boylan, pp. 215–16.

Introduction to the Original

LET me give the reader a somewhat rasping jolt in the very beginning—and get that out of the way.

I am a patient in a "State Hospital"—as insane asylums are now called in an attempt to lessen the harsh impression created by the designation formerly in use.

I am locked in, like the other patients. I live the life they live. As I am one of them, I am the recipient of their confidences; the target for the unrepressed revealing of their quirks, obsessions and delusions. I see them when they are not on guard.

Is it egotism, then, for me to believe that I know my strange associates from a viewpoint which others, even the physicians in charge, cannot have? The physicians and attendants know them from the viewpoint of the observing scientist or of the curbing and disciplinary authority set over them. In spite of sincere efforts to understand them, the officials must always look down on the mentally afflicted from a height, an attitude which those in charge of the insane cannot avoid or change.

Also I frankly believe that I am in a position to see the officials, the conduct of the institution, and the attitude of the public from a viewpoint which neither those who must control and guard the aberrated nor the average layman can get—the viewpoint of one of the patients.

If I can give the matter-of-fact, every-day men and women on the "great outside" some true conception of what goes on within the minds of the inmates of a state hospital for the insane, and of the attitude of those into whose charge they are given, then I will have accomplished one purpose of this story of my long, long months "On the Receiving Ward."

To do this it is necessary for me, first, to erase the fantastic mental picture which the average person has of such an institution and its inmates. I must banish the "madhouse" conception which springs into the uninformed mind at the mere mention of an insane asylum. Then, if the reader maintains an open and receptive mind, I may be able to give him a fairly true conception of the insane.

I can do this best by giving an intimate picturization of the events which have taken place since first I was checked in on the receiving ward, of my treatment at the hands of physicians, attendants and visitors and by portraying faithfully the life of my associates, their modes of thought, their hopes, their fears and their philosophies.

Yes, their philosophies; for even in insane asylums men and women have their philosophies.

I am acutely aware that, with some readers, its very realism, unadorned, will militate against the story. It contains no tense situations, no harrowing suspenses, no smashing climaxes. It is innocent of literary nonsense. It is too conscientiously true for that.

But for that large part of the American reading public which takes pride in knowing unusual facts, readably presented; and for those who may be concerned with any of the 350,000 inmates of state asylums, I hope this story will have keen interest and lasting informative value.

Also, I am acutely aware that, exactly as I have taken the liberty of judging my associates by their thought processes, my readers will take impish delight in figuratively prying open my cranium and uncompromisingly judging me by my own psychological standards.

Through this receiving ward flow all the men patients who are committed to the institution. Not only are they received here but they are kept here during a period of observation; a time in which they can be studied, and the officials can determine to what specific wards they should be assigned permanently. Whether they come in with their commitment papers marked "violent" or merely "depressed"; whether they are raving or appear to be in full possession of their reasoning and comprehensive faculties, they are kept for a time on the receiving ward. Those who are exceptionally rational and amenable often are permanently retained on the ward.

Thus a picture of life on the receiving ward during the long time that I have been here will give an excellent cross section of that in the entire institution; the ward having harbored during that time all classes of patients, from the madman of popular conception to the helpless old man in his natural dotage who has been shunted into the asylum by heartless relatives, or by the busy, unconsidering public.

Oh yes, Smug Ladies and Gentlemen; some of these do come in.

Prologue

THEY are taking Barney Murray to one of the violent wards. He has just been led out of this ward between two stalwart attendants, who held his arms pinioned behind his back as they hustled him determinedly down the stairs and along the broad concrete walk which leads to Ward J. They know just how to hold him to keep him from being able to fight back. That is a part of their business.

We other patients on the receiving ward are sorry to see Murray go. He has been such a likable fellow; merry, pleasant, considerate and thoughtful of others—and he never bothered one of us by telling us his troubles. He was such a very likable fellow.

Now he has gone violent, and they are taking him to Ward J.

Perhaps it would have been better for him if he had told some of us about his troubles, even if it did make us irritable and impatient. Perhaps he kept them too closely locked up in his own brain, and brooded on them at night. And then perhaps he listened too much to the weird delusions and warped vagaries of others. Who knows?

We did not gather round and tell Murray good-bye. We do not do that when they are taken to Ward J. We see so many go that way—after they have been locked in here for awhile. We are quite apathetic about it. It is just a part of the life here. We do not know who will be next.

We have known for three days that Murray was "going off." His merry cheerfulness disappeared. He moped around moodily by himself, with that queer light of irrationality growing in his eyes. This morning he cracked.

He began talking to himself. He soaked a towel in water and tied it about his head. He gathered all the paper he could find or beg, tore it into fine bits and kept sifting these bits through his fingers as though he were mixing powders of different kinds.

He told us he was making a preparation to kill the cockroaches in the ward.

"It's easy to make when you know how," he told me. "I've been working on it for a long time, and I just learned how to do it. Look here; isn't this easy?" He snatched up the sheet of paper on which I was writing, tore it into tiny bits and sifted the bits through his fingers several times. Then he handed them to me. "Save that for the doctors," he said. "They will want to know how to do it."

Then the cloud which had come over his mind took a twist toward destructiveness. He stripped off his clothes and tied the outer garments in numerous hard knots. He tore his underwear into shreds. The attendants came and got him, put another suit of underwear on him and locked him in his room. He shredded the second suit of underwear, did the same to his bed sheets and started breaking up the chair in his room.

So they are taking him to Ward J.

I can see him through my window, as the attendants march him along, holding his arms twisted up behind his back so that he can not fight. There he goes, up the broad steps to Ward J. That's the way so many of them go after they have been here awhile. And he was such a likable fellow. He never bothered me with his troubles.

I turn back to my work—not my regular duties on the ward—I am through with them for day—but to a careful re-reading of what I have ploddingly written during the long months that I have been here. I have been studying it, trying to see it as others would see it.

I have been a long time in writing it, doggedly plugging away at it day after day, dragging the words to express it out of a mind which was ineffably weary, suddenly reluctant to respond.

I have written it whenever I could find snatches of time between carrying out my regular ward duties and continually but diplomatically shooing out of my room other patients who wanted to tell me, irrationally but impassionedly and often, how they are being held here against their will, when they are "all right and should go home."

And now I am re-reading what I have written. I am asking myself in all sincerity, "Will I be able to get across to the mind of the reader a true and clean-edged conception of the story I am trying to tell?"

Not by what I have told, perhaps. It would take a clearer mind and a defter stroke than I possess to paint such a picture through the medium of printed lines.

Shall I tear up these pages, produced in the midst of mental turmoil, in my own mind and in all the minds round about me. Shall I wait for a time of clearer and less disturbed perception before trying to write the story?

No; I will leave it just as I have written it from day to day. I believe the reader will be able to read between my plodding lines; to trace from chapter to chapter the gradual lifting of the torpid heaviness of mind out of which I have had to drag myself, even as I wrote; and to see, in the telling of the story, a surer touch and a clearer judgment as the months here have passed over my head.

And I believe that in the conception he thus creates for himself in his own mind he will get a true picture of life inside a hospital for the insane, of my associates in such a hospital, and of the woman who refuses to forget me, and my still continuing struggles to retain and bulwark my sanity while I am reshaping and rebuilding my mental and moral manhood.

BEHIND THE
DOOR OF DELUSION

CHAPTER I

Checked In

THE deputy sheriff who had brought me from my home city ushered me into the big office building of the institution, and along a hallway to a central room, where a large, spectacled man sat at a desk.

"Good evening, Doctor, I have brought you another," boomed the deputy sheriff, who has charge of transporting all the insane from my own county to the hospital.

The doctor turned to me without a word. There was an embarrassing pause as he looked me over critically. As would be natural under like circumstances but different surroundings, I introduced myself and offered my hand. Immediately I realized that I had done something wrong. The look which the doctor gave me simply set me back on my heels. My hand remained untaken.

Then I realized with a shock that this was not a meeting of two gentlemen on a plane of equality. In the eyes of the man before me I was just another insane patient, duly committed and now awaiting his orders. I had stepped far off my own plane when I expected him to acknowledge my introduction of myself.

I know that my face flushed hotly as my mind assimilated the fact that I was no longer a widely known citizen of my own home city, a welcomed speaker at luncheon clubs and an active figure in civic affairs; I now was only one of the patients in a state hospital for the insane, just one of the submerged two thousand, and I had had my first lesson in institutional discipline.

Well, I would not make another mistake of the kind, I told myself. I would learn my place and keep it. I knew I must step carefully and let closer acquaintance and my conduct recommend me to those now in charge of me, and who would judge me by my actions.

The doctor entered my name, age, height and the name of the county from which I came, on a blank form. A wide shouldered attendant and another man were waiting, and took me in charge. I was led down a long concrete walk to another of the large, sombre brick buildings.

I noted that both of the men kept hold of my arms. I smiled rather wryly at the realization that they feared I might make a "break" for freedom. Again I felt a sinking sensation at the thought that to them, also, I was just one of the patients, and on the level which all patients in an insane asylum must occupy.

Later I was to learn just how quickly these men, long experienced in judging incoming patients, are able to distinguish between those capable of conducting themselves according to ordinary standards and those who require sharp disciplinary repression. But when a man is first received it is absolutely necessary that he be handled with caution until the attendants and officials have had an opportunity to study him under many different conditions. It often happens that a patient who is quiet and tractable when received will suddenly suffer a delusion and become wildly uncontrollable, without warning.

I was led into the building which was to be my home, for nobody knows how long; through a ground floor ward where half a hundred men, many of them in the nondescript clothing supplied by the state, peered at me curiously and, I thought, half furtively. I had the feeling that I was some wild animal newly arrived at the zoo and was being looked over with distrust and suspicion by those animals already there.

We climbed a flight of steps, the white coated attendant unlocked a heavy oaken door and I was ushered inside the receiving ward. A key grated in a lock as the heavy door was secured. I had become one of those locked in.

Another white coated attendant came briskly forward. "Come right in here," he said as he led me into a large, steamy and smelly bath-room where one of the two tubs had been filled, evidently in expectation of my arrival. "Undress and take a bath," I was ordered. The tone was not particularly unkindly but there was a timbre in it which showed that the attendant intended to be obeyed without question or demurrer. I obeyed.

While I was undressing, the attendant was busy asking me questions and entering the answers on a blank form. The door of the bath-room was open into the long hall, and inmates crowded it to get a look at the new patient. I squirmed, mentally, as they eyed me. The attendant looked up, sharply. "Clear the hall," he shouted. The men reluctantly melted away. But the attraction of looking over a new patient was too strong. Furtively they found their way back, presently, while the attendant was examining my stripped body for marks or scars.

As he looked me over a young man in the garb of a patient wrote down the location and description of each scar. The whole thing dropped my drooping spirits still lower. I was being "tabbed" just like a prisoner. Then it burst on me again that in truth I was a prisoner; not in the sense that I had committed any crime, but that the law said that I must be kept locked up. The realization cut, and cut deeply.

I bathed myself. The room reeked of steam and strong, smelly soap. How different from the tiled bath-rooms and mildly scented soaps that I had used for years. The men peering in at me as I went through my ablutions made it even worse. Well, I must become accustomed to it.

The attendant came, bringing a suit of coarse cotton underwear with long sleeves and legs. I had worn athletic underwear, summer and winter, since such garments first came on the market. But I climbed into that shapeless suit with a smile, as though I liked it. I was trying to learn my place; trying to follow my cues. "This way," ordered the attendant. I was led through a large and sunny gathering room or "day hall" into an even larger room where beds—row on row of them—neatly made up, were waiting. "Take this one. It will be your bed until you are changed," the attendant said. I climbed in and pulled up the sheet and blanket. The attendant perched himself on the foot of the bedstead and faced me.

As he studied me, I studied him. He was a very blond young man, not more than twenty-six years of age. He was slender. He looked more like a man recently out of college than one set to control approximately sixty partially irresponsible men. But he had the indescribable air of a man who has authority and is accustomed to exercising it.

A somewhat similar air is attained by policemen, sheriffs and other peace officers, but there is a distinctive difference. The better attendants, being of a higher mental type than the average policeman, and being under watchful supervision, have little of the offensiveness and suggestion of brutality which so many policemen acquire.

There are some brutal attendants in most insane asylums, I have since learned, reliably. But usually they are weeded out as soon as they are detected in any brutality by the hospital authorities. I have never found but one on this ward. From patients on other wards I have learned of some rough handling of patients by attendants who have since been discharged.

But personally I have never witnessed an actual case of intentional brutality. But as this attendant sat on the foot of my bed and faced me I knew that he not only expected to be obeyed but that he fully intended to be obeyed implicitly.

"Well," he began, "I am not going to attempt to fill your mind full of the rules and regulations of this hospital. If I undertook to tell you all about them you probably would not remember half of them. But you can get along all right by remembering this one thing. Just conduct yourself as a man. Be a man at all times and you will not run against many of the regulations. And whenever you do happen to do something which is not permitted you'll find it out, all right, and remember it.

"There will be many things here that you do not like. You will have to do some things that you do not want to do. But the thing to do is just to be a man and do them, whether they please you or not. We easily can tell when you willfully break a rule, and when you go wrong because you simply don't know.

"Now you are not the type to break rules willfully. You will try to conduct yourself properly."

He must have caught the look on my face for he grinned and said: "I know I am young in age but I am old in this work. I have been in it for several years. I have served on almost every ward in this hospital. I have learned to size up patients mighty quickly. Now you are to stay in bed; that is your first order. Stay there all day tomorrow. I may want you to stay there the next day. If so, just be patient and stay.

"You may think you are all right mentally. Very probably you do. Most of them do. But at least you are locked up. That means you must show us the stuff you are made of; prove to us you are all right.

"The first night or two here you may not sleep much. About forty men sleep in this room. It's a bedlam sometimes. But in two or three nights you will find that you can sleep right through it."

That was my initiation as a patient in an asylum. It gave me another impression to add to those which I had already acquired. I was weak physically; my nerves were unstrung and my mind was deadly weary. But this impression sank in. "How different from the treatment usually pictured as handed out in a madhouse."

The attendant went about his duties. I lay in bed, more than wide awake, my mind whirling under a tumbling wave of thoughts. Other patients stole to the door of the dormitory and peeped in to get another look at me. To avoid their eyes I looked over the room in which I was lying.

There were three or four other men in bed, although it was only late afternoon. I rightly guessed that these were other new patients, or inmates who were not able to be up and about. In the bed immediately beside mine was a rather small man with wild, staring eyes which incessantly darted everywhere, yet seemed to see nothing.

He mumbled to himself and made strange noises in his throat. He had kicked the covers off and at times he writhed and twisted his body into grotesque shapes. His very nearness made me shudder. Yet my greatest reaction was pity—pity for a mind so self-tortured.

Finally his twistings threw him out of bed. He struck the floor with a solid thump. An attendant came briskly in. Several of the inmates, without being called, came at once to assist him. The writhing patient was lifted back into bed.

"Get a strait-jacket," the attendant told one of the patients. I stiffened. I had heard, vaguely, of strait-jackets. In my mind they were instruments of torture; at least of punishment. My hazy idea was that they were much like some of the torture devices of the Spanish Inquisition.

The patient came back, bringing a canvas jacket. My jaw dropped, for it certainly did not come up to my expectations. It looked decidedly harmless. In a moment or two the man was clothed in it, down to the waist; it came only to the waist line.

His arms were now encased in sleeves of heavy canvas, closed at the ends to cover the hands. Cords were attached to the closed ends of the sleeves so that when the patient's arms were folded they could be held in that position by tying the cords behind his back. He now was helpless to scratch or otherwise hurt himself, but he had the freedom of his lower limbs. The strait-jacket was only a device to protect the patient from himself.

Lifted back into bed, the jacketed patient was strapped to the bedstead. But the bonds were wide bands of heavy bed ticking which would neither chafe him nor prevent his resting. However they would prevent him from throwing himself out of the bed upon the hard floor, and perhaps suffering nasty bruises.

I turned away in order not to see his twistings and writhings. As he was now secured, the attendants and patients paid no further attention to him for the time being. But I lay there through that long, long afternoon, forced to listen to his mumblings, meaningless and guttural, high pitched and querulous by turns. And he was almost within reach of me.

A man came into the room carrying a tray and a tin bucket of milk. He came to my bed and handed me a tin plate, piled high with food and topped with a very thick slice of bread, as large as the crown of a hat. Next he handed me a tin cup of milk, poured from the bucket.

I looked at my plate. There was plenty of food there, all right. In fact there was entirely too much. But its arrangement and scrambled condition did not appeal to my weakened appetite. The black-eyed peas had become somewhat mixed up with the boiled rice, and a dab of mashed potatoes was an island, entirely surrounded by noodles. To a man whose usual dinner begins with a good salad and ends with a dessert and black coffee, the conglomeration did not look tempting.

I drank the milk, noting that it tasted very thin. I dabbed at the mashed potatoes with a table spoon. They had not brought me any knife or fork. I learned why, later.

Noting my failure to eat, the man who had brought the food said sharply, "You had better eat. You'll get strong quicker."

"I believe that I don't care for dinner," I said weakly. "Dinner?" was the retort: "Up here, fellow, this meal is supper." I felt rebuked.

The man turned to the patient in the strait-jacket. He loosened the cloth bands, lifted the patient to a sitting posture and fed him. It was not accomplished easily. Several times the patient slumped down in bed. He would not open his mouth until sharply ordered to do so, then his mouth would fly open as though propelled by a spring. A spoonful of food would be popped into it before he had time to close it. Finally the feeding was finished.

Slowly, slowly night came on. Out in the day room the many inmates showed signs of restlessness. Suddenly an attendant shouted, "Bed time." Then the bedlam of which I had been forewarned, began.

Into the dormitory swarmed the nearly two score men who slept there. They were talking and laughing, in a dozen keys.

Volleys of "Goodnights" were being shouted across the room. One man, with whom the action seemed to be an obsession, was attempting to say goodnight to every other man in the room, calling each by name and insisting on a reply. Gradually the men undressed, placed their folded clothes on the foot of the beds and rolled beneath the covers.

Slowly the sounds of the day ceased, but other sounds took their place. Snores arose. Stertorous breathings added an undertone. Over in a far corner a patient who continually talks to himself was emitting whispered conversations with an imaginary listener, and the whispers had a penetrating quality which I have found nowhere else.

In the bed next to mine the man in the strait-jacket twisted and pulled at the bands which held him. He swore horribly, at first under his breath, but later aloud.

An attendant came and administered a mild sedative. But, as is sometimes the case with those who are violently insane, the sedative failed to quiet the man. For an hour more he mouthed and cursed. The attendant administered another sedative without noticeable result. He called one of the other patients. Together the two picked up the bed, jacketed patient and all, and carried it out into the day room.

This reduced the disturbance. But since the door between the two rooms was open so that the attendant could keep an eye on all that went on in both rooms, and since I was feverishly awake, I could still hear the man's ravings all through the night. And that night seemed to be uncounted ages long.

Just when my screaming nerves seemed as though they could last but little longer without breaking under the strain, the night attendant came briskly into the dormitory and switched on the lights. "All out," he shouted sharply. And in a twinkling the men were rolling out of their beds or sitting up on them, putting on their clothes.

A glance at the unshaded windows showed me that it still was dark outside. I had no idea of the time. My watch, in fact everything that I had brought with me, had been taken away when I was first undressed and put to bed. But it needed no watch to tell me that the patients were getting up at an hour but little later than that at which I, the usual 1930 model night-hawk, was accustomed to going to bed. As my first full day in the asylum started I wondered if I would ever become accustomed to going to bed shortly after dusk and getting up before even the first gray streak of dawn.

The men, each one grabbing a towel from beneath his mattress, were rushing out to an unseen lavatory and coming back shortly with faces washed and hair combed. Some one switched on a radio in the day room and a program began coming in.

Then a bell tinkled somewhere. The men lined up, two by two, rather irregularly. An attendant unlocked a door leading into the interior of the building and the patients marched off to breakfast. My breakfast was brought to me by the same man who had so sharply advised me to eat, the evening before. In spite of the weakened condition in which I had arrived I found that my long fast had made me slightly hungry. The food probably looked just as scrambled as it did the night before, at "supper," but it looked somewhat different in my eyes. I fingered the heavy table-spoon gingerly, but I ate.

And thus began my first full day in the asylum;—a day in which I was to see much and learn much that I could have learned in no other way.

CHAPTER II

THE LONELY DRAG

IT was not the attendants who taught me most about the insane, or about the men in the hospitals who are not insane. Nor was it the physicians. I myself was an inmate and the other inmates accepted me as one of themselves and gave me their confidences. With apologies to Kipling—I learned about patients from them.

I lay in bed, that first morning that I spent behind asylum walls. The mental turmoil of the night had left my already weakened nervous system quivering. My mind was in a condition bordering on a daze.

About me the daytime activities of the hospital hummed. All the work was done by the patients. There was little detailed supervision by the attendants, although they were here, there and everywhere all the time. One of them would shout an order and the patients, stolidly and mechanically, would carry it out. They seemed to have been trained in the work until it had become almost automatic.

"Chairs out," the head attendant shouted. Lines of patients carried the chairs, benches and tables out of the big day room. "Floor gang; get busy," the attendant roared. Men swept the floor with plodding deliberateness. "Polishers out." A group of patients began polishing the hardwood floors with "polishers" made of heavy blocks of wood, covered with strips of old blankets.

Certain patients were making up the beds. They did it with a neatness which would shame many of the maids in good hotels. Some carefully mopped the concrete floors of the hallway, bathroom and lavatory. Some wiped off doors and other woodwork with oiled cloths. And some, formed in double file and accompanied by an attendant, were marched out of the ward. These, I afterward learned, worked in the art department, bakery, the store, or other departments of the institution.

But none of this activity was for me, on that first morning. I had been told to lie in bed. And I could not have got up if I had wanted to do so. I had no clothing except the coarse cotton underwear in which I was lying. My clothes had been taken away. I was feverish. My mouth felt hot and dry. The weakened physical and nervous condition in which I had arrived and the mental strain I had since undergone were affecting me. I was very thirsty. I hoped that an attendant would come near my bed so that I could ask for a drink of water. I am tempted to believe that men whose minds are somewhat clouded become unconsciously psychic. They seem to read the wants of others in their position. Certain it is that as I longed for water one of the patients approached my bed.

He was one of those poor fellows whom a nervous affliction has distorted physically. The muscles of his neck had contracted and drawn his head backward until his face was looking almost straight upward. His fingers were drawn into tightly clenched knots. He did not seem to be able to close his mouth, and his upper lip was drawn back until all of his upper teeth showed. He walked only with a twisted motion. Yet his mind seemed to be fairly clear.

He was trying to smile. Out of that twisted mouth came the question—"D-don't you w-want a d-wink of w-water?"

"Yes, indeed I do; thank you," I answered; and he shuffled painfully off, to return a few moments later with a brimming tin cup, held between the flats of his hands. I drank thirstily. And I had a changed and more generous opinion of that youth; he was scarcely more than a boy. He was terribly afflicted. I previously had felt almost a repugnance when I looked at him. But he was doing his best to be thoughtful and helpful.

Several times during that long day patients came to my bed. They wanted to know if there was anything they could do for me. Most of them seemed to be genuinely sympathetic and anxious to be helpful although some of them were almost offensively curious about me. They all talked to me of their own affairs and a few, with a slightly shamefaced air, told me why they were committed to the hospital. "I guess I went a little off," was the way they put it.

They never failed to ask why I "had come" and if I had a family, and every one of them invariably wound up with a question which seems to be foremost in the minds of every asylum inmate, whether sane or insane—"how long I expected" to stay.

The answer to that question none of us who are locked in can know. God! If we only could. There is no definite "term" for those incarcerated in an asylum. We never know when we are "going home."

In spite of the thoughtfulness of some of the patients the day dragged out slowly—exhaustingly slowly. During the afternoon an attendant came in accompanied by several of the patients. The man who had been placed in the strait-jacket the previous night was partially dressed and conducted out of the ward. I asked one of the patients where he was being taken. "To the Hydro," was the brief answer.

I was interested. Just what was the Hydro, I wondered. I asked the question. "Oh, that's where they pack 'em in water or in ice. It makes 'em sweat and helps the violent ones; some of 'em it cures," my informant replied. I was to learn more about the Hydro later and get less misleading information regarding this treatment for certain forms and stages of insanity.

During all that day no attendant came near me. Neither of the two on duty spoke to me or asked if there was anything I desired. Apparently they left this to the older patients.

But several times, during the day, I caught the attendant who was in charge gazing at me in dispassionate mental appraisal.

Evening came. A new inmate arrived. A patient told me that they were coming in at a rate of more than fifty each month.

The new man strenuously objected to taking a bath—but he had to take one, nevertheless. "If you were the governor of the state and happened to be sent here you would have to take a bath, just the same," one of the attendants told him. "And if you were the governor himself you could not get out in less than thirty days." I have learned that this is literally true.

The latest arrival was placed in the bed next to mine. He was not violent in the least, but he was an epileptic and he had three convulsions during the night. Again I could not sleep. His quivering nervousness seemed to he transmitted to me. Certainly it made me nervous and excitable. Worn, nerve-jangled and tossing, I wearily asked myself, "Why, Oh why do they put two new patients in adjoining beds?"

Later observation has shown the that the attendants do make an effort to avoid placing close together those patients who will rasp each other's nerves too harshly. I have also learned how impossible it is for them to accomplish this under present methods of handling the insane. The world has not reached the stage where peace of mind or freedom from nerve-wrecking contacts is considered as having a place in the treatment or alleviation of insanity. The patients are crowded—massed—together where the mental quirks of each continually and inevitably tear and wear at the weakened minds of the others.

My second night was as horribly tenuous and exhausting as the first. Another day passed and I was still kept in bed. The ward physician, on his hurried, daily round, gave me a searching look and passed on. The attendants paid no apparent attention to me.

Even the patients who had visited my bed the previous day seemed to have lost a part of their interest in me. There were more recent arrivals to feed their curiosity.

But on the third morning the physician stopped beside my bed and asked, "Well, how do you feel?" I tried to keep my voice steady and controlled as I answered that I was feeling very much better. The physician said something in an undertone to the attendant who accompanied him, then the two moved on to other beds.

A few minutes later the attendant came back. "Would you like to get up?" he asked. I am afraid that I was not able to keep the eagerness out of my voice as I answered that I would be very thankful to be permitted to do so. "Come on," said the attendant, and I followed him into the clothes-storage room.

But, alack! I was not dressed in my own clothing. Near-shapeless "state" garments were doled out to me. I hesitatingly asked if I could not have my own clothing. "Certainly not," was the reply. "They have been sent to the sterilizer to be cleaned and disinfected. You can have them when they get back. These clothes have been used but they have been cleaned since that. Don't worry about them." I straightened my wry face, started dressing and soon was arrayed in a much faded blue denim shirt, equally faded cotton trousers, heavy and coarse cotton socks of the "hayseed" type and color, and a cotton sweater of no particular color whatever, and which could not boast a single button.

When I was dressed I went over to a mirror which hung on the wall. One look in it—and at first I wanted to find the fabled caves where the walls fall on you and hide you. Then the saving humor of the situation came to my aid and I was able to manage a chuckle.

The melting pot of the receiving ward had functioned perfectly. With a three days' growth of beard on my face and dressed in those clothes I was an exact counterpart of the other patients who were dressed in the same way. A visitor, passing through the ward, would have seen nothing to set me apart in any way from the rest of them. Clothes do make the man, so far as the casual observer is concerned. At least they express and accentuate his personality and station in life. On the receiving ward the casual visitor could not distinguish the ex-banker from the former ditch-digger. And the state hospitals house many men of both classes, sitting on the same benches, carrying out much the same duties, dreading the slow passage of time in the same way and both acquiring the pallor which comes only from long confinement within doors.

Patients are permitted to wear their own clothes, if they have them. But this necessitates the expense of laundry and cleaning, and the replacement of the clothes when they wear out. And money is scarcer in an asylum ward than—well, than cotton stockings in Hollywood.

Some few of the patients receive small remittances from "home" but a large majority must depend on the tiny amounts which they can earn by doing little services for the more fortunate ones.

They shine shoes, clean up rooms and do light laundry work for the others, in most instances. And a puny dime will induce any one of them to wash a shirt and underwear and a week's supply of socks and handkerchiefs. Try that on your laundry.

I felt that I was being granted a favor when I was permitted to get out of bed and dress. Half an hour later I was willing to concede that I had jumped out of the frying pan into the fire. I was told to go into the day room and sit down.

The chairs and settees ranged along the walls looked comfortable enough. And they were—for a time. Most of them were occupied by patients; one or two reading, the rest just sitting. There was little conversation, and that in subdued tones. At a table in the center of the room sat an attendant who was busy filling out what appeared to be report forms; nevertheless his eyes traveled continually about the room. I somehow felt that I was being watched, and I was restless under the scrutiny.

So I sat there, just like the others. I had nothing to read; I had nothing to do but chew my scrambled thoughts. Soon I was squirming in my chair. Time was dragging, dragging, dragging.

Restlessly I looked about for some one to whom I could talk. No one near me seemed to pay the slightest attention to me. The patients just sat there, silent, staring into space. Some of them looked sullen. Others looked just vacant-minded.

Then I noticed that none of the chairs were occupied by any of the men who had visited me while I was in bed. I had become somewhat acquainted with several of them. Finally I happened to look down the long hallway which led out of one side of the day room. Off of it on either side doors opened into small rooms. In the hallway I recognized two or three of the patients with whom I had become acquainted. I saw in them an opportunity for conversation, and anything would help that awful monotony. I rose eagerly and started to walk toward them. And, exactly as the charge attendant had predicted, I "found out" that I had made another false move.

"Here," called the attendant sharply. "Where are you going?" I weakly replied that I was "just going down the hall." "Oh no you are not," the attendant said. "You are not allowed down there. Go back to your seat." Meekly I went back to the wearing monotony of my chair.

Sitting still becomes wearing under any circumstances, but if you are compelled to sit still it is far worse. It can become almost a twitching torture, particularly to a nervous person. And for its sheer worst form let me commend enforced sitting still on a ward of an insane asylum.

To make it worse I could see other men in the hall, laughing and talking. I felt badly militated against and both hurt and angry because I was not permitted to do the same thing.

Then one of the men who had been out in the hallway came into the day hall and sat down beside me. And again I felt that these men are in some degree psychic. The patient immediately began to tell me about the rules of the ward.

"You're new here, ain't you? Well you'll have some trouble finding your way about for a few days. It ain't so bad, though, and you'll catch on. There don't seem to be much the matter with you, anyway. Where're you from?" I told him, briefly.

"Well, you see those rooms down the hall? They belong to the parole men, mostly, though some of 'em belong to men who are not paroled but have been here a long time and haven't much the matter with 'em. You have to get a room order from the doctor to get one. You new fellows and all the fellows who haven't got rooms are not allowed to go down that hall farther than to the door of the card room. It's a good rule. It keeps some of these bugs from coming bulging into your room and bothering you and maybe stealing something. I don't want some of these nuts ever coming into my room at all; not the real crazy ones. And you can't always tell. How long do you expect to be here?"

I sadly told him that I did not know.

"Well you don't look like there is much the matter with you. They'll probably let you have a parole after you have been here sixty or ninety days. Still you never can tell. But maybe you can get a room before very long. Then it won't be so bad."

The mention of the card room had caught my ear instantly. It offered relief from the deadly monotony of sitting still and quiet. I asked where it was and if I would be permitted in it. "It's right down the hall there, just this side of the living rooms. Yeah, you can go to it after you been here a few days. Better ask the attendant, though, before you try it. You are new here and they don't know much about you. They got to study you. Then they'll let you go, all right. There's cards there and checkers and one of the boys has a chess set. They all help to pass the time," my volunteer informant replied.

"Have they sent you to the clinic yet? Well they'll let you know when they want you and after the doctors have examined you they will know more about you and it won't be so bad. You don't look like you had much the matter with you. You'll get along all right. The first thirty days is the worst; that is, until you get stir fever."

I groped at the words. "What is stir fever?" I asked.

The man eyed me in frank disdain. "Say, what business are you in?" he asked. I answered that I was a newspaper man.

"You in the newspaper game and don't know what stir fever is? Well after you've been locked up long enough you'll know," was the haughty retort. "You'll get tired of being locked up so long, then you'll have bad spells of restlessness and you'll sit around gloomy all day wondering how to get out of here. Sure you will. All of 'em do. Most of 'em try it."

His tone made me blush for my ignorance.

"When you want exercise you can go out on the porch and walk. You'll learn to do it. It's good for you," he pursued in a more conciliatory tone.

I had noticed the porch. It ran along one side of the big day hall and was much like an ordinary sun porch except that its unglassed window-spaces were protected by light iron bars, arranged like lattice work. Except for these bars the porch was open to the searching winter breezes. Men were tramping up and down it, singly or in pairs. They walked rapidly but stolidly as though the exercise were a serious duty. Under the circumstances that is exactly what it was.

While the talkative patient continued to rattle on a hidden bell rang. There was an immediate rush for the door leading down stairs. An attendant unlocked the door and led the irregular double file of patients down two flights of steps to the dining room. Accustomed to good elevators I felt that that walk down two flights of stairs was quite a task. I since have learned to bless those steps. They give me more exercise and a relief from the hard floors of the ward.

If you think that hard, uncarpeted floors are not distinctly tiring, just ask a waiter or the floor walker of a second rate department store. And their working day seldom is more than eight hours long. The average patient in an insane asylum never gets to walk on anything but concrete or hardwood, year in and year out, and he gets up at 5 o'clock in the morning and goes to bed at 8 o'clock at night.

As the patients reached the dining room each one went to his own place at the tables. No one had assigned me a place so I walked over to an attendant and asked him where I should sit. To my surprise he seized me roughly by the arm. "Look here," he said, "When you want to know anything you call me. Don't you go to walking all over the dining room again. Do you hear?"

He kept hold of my arm and escorted me to a vacant place. During dinner one of the patients told me why walking about the dining room is not permitted. It would give too great an opportunity for some patient to filch and conceal a knife. Cases of this kind have occurred here, I was told.

A knife, fork and spoon is put beside each plate but they are collected before the patients leave the room and each man must account for all of his table utensils. The men who collect them must account for the full number when they turn them in at the kitchen.

The meal cheered me somewhat. I now had a plate, teacup and knife and fork, which I had not had when eating in bed. The food was served in large dishes and I could help myself, thus avoiding scrambling the food. The menu was as limited and drab as before and the food just as badly cooked. But it is surprising how much better black-eyed peas, potatoes, bread and syrup taste when they are not jumbled together in a soppy mass.

During the afternoon several of the patients continued to give me information about the institution, its rules, the other patients and themselves. One would come and sit beside me and talk for awhile, then he would suddenly get up without apparent reason and go somewhere else. But gradually I acquired considerable information that I needed.

I was warned about drinking from the tin cups without first scalding them out, as many of the patients are suffering from loathsome social diseases. "You'd be surprised to know how many of the fellows have cases, especially when they first come in," my informant said. "Some of them are just rotting away with it. And they have other diseases; and some are lousy. Just scald out your cup. There is a hot water tap right beside the cups. But don't get careless. Better try to get you a cup of your own, if you can."

He wasted that admonition about not getting careless. His description made my flesh crawl. And I shuddered at the thought that I would have to use the same cups as the afflicted men, even if they had been scalded. I did not feel very comfortable, either, at the thought that the clothes I had on and the linens of my bed might have been used previously by a man who was just "rotting away with it."

I knew, of course, that the hospital authorities certainly must take every precaution to avoid infecting other patients, but just the same the thoughts of the possibilities gave me a decided cringing.

My companion was not through with his course of instruction and I was even more anxious to learn than he was to impart. "Be careful who you chum with, up here," he warned. "Some of these bugs here don't know anything. If you pay any attention to them at all they'll just hang themselves on to you and you can't get rid of them at all. They'll run you crazy. Now, some of the fellows are pretty sensible. You just learn who they are and hang onto them. There don't seem to be much the matter with you; not just now, anyway."

I was to learn that this was excellent advice. Also I tried to learn who were the men who were "pretty sensible." I soon felt that I could be fairly accurate in my judgment after the first extended conversation with a patient.

But I made some woeful mistakes. I was to learn that a patient who apparently is in sound mind most of the time can suddenly suffer a paroxysm of wild hallucinations and become thoroughly and irresponsibly insane or even dangerously violent, then after a period, return to an apparently normal state. One of the older attendants here expressed this to me, characteristically, later.

"Some of the fellows who, when they are themselves, are the nicest and quietest and do whatever you tell them to, are the most dangerous when they have a spell. And when a man is unusually quiet for a few days, watch him. He is usually getting ready to start something—although some of them fly off when you least expect it. We have to watch everybody, all the time."

I have seen this graphically illustrated many, many times.

During that first day that I was out of bed I learned what is meant by a "parole man." He is a patient who is believed to have recovered, or one whom the authorities believe can be trusted to have the freedom of the hospital grounds, under certain restrictions. Such patients are given "grounds roles." They have the wonderful advantage of outdoor exercise and a feeling of partial freedom. Also they are given certain responsibilities.

It is usually the parole men who assist the attendants in handling other patients; in bathing them, conducting them to the dining room, and restraining them physically when this is required. But this is not always true. Some of the most incurably insane give very valuable assistance in restraining violent men, if permitted to do so.

My intimate association with the insane, daily for month after month, convinces me that nearly every insane man believes that he is more sane than the other inmates. With a majority of them the more insane they are the more firmly they are convinced that there is nothing wrong with them. It is only the better patients, those who are most nearly sane, who will acknowledge that they are, or have been, "a little off." I have seen epileptics, coming out of a half hour convulsion, swear heatedly that they had had no convulsion, and become violently angry at the men who carried them to their beds or otherwise assisted them.

Yet some of these very fellows will be the first to assist another epileptic who is in a convulsion.

But, directly contrary to the usual belief, I have found my insane associates to be pretty accurate judges of the degree of insanity of other patients. One man here, who is classed as permanently insane, looks over every new patient who is brought in and immediately gives me his opinion of the new man's case. "Did you see the new man?" he will say. "He is as crazy as a bedbug. He never will get to go home." Or he may say, "That man is not much crazy. He'll make a good man on the ward." I have not yet seen his judgment fail to be correct. Other patients are just as accurate in their judgment of the degree of insanity of the regular inmates of the ward.

But in the next breath after telling me which patients on the ward are badly insane and which are not, they may start in to tell me that they are expecting to be discharged next week, or to give me elaborate but impracticable details of what they plan doing when they go home.

Even on that first day I began to sense this. Two or three of the patients gave me a very accurate list of the men who were "pretty sensible." Their judgment was better than mine; I made some bad mistakes in picking out the more rational patients.

That first day finally drew to a close. Night time came, and with it the attendant's stentorian call of "Bed time." I undressed and crawled wearily between the sheets. Blessed relief. I was so worn out from the past sleepless nights that I immediately went to sleep. I found that the charge attendant had been right when he predicted that sooner or later I would be able to sleep in spite of the bedlam.

The man who talks continually was whispering just as penetratingly as ever. The scores of sorted snores and stertorous breathings were just as loud. One patient was mouthing unintelligible mutterings as I placed my head on the pillow.

One moment I was flinchingly conscious of each separate, grating discordance in that cacophony of wheezings and whisperings. The next, and I was dropping, through leagues and leagues of space, into a softly enfolding, grateful oblivion. I slept,—unconscious of it all.

CHAPTER III

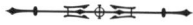

OUR SANE INSANE

A WEEK had dragged its weary, torturing and tortuous way to an end since I was locked in on the receiving ward. I had not been called before the mental clinic. I had nothing to do to occupy and relieve my mind and keep me from brooding, except to learn all that I could and catch a conversation where and when I might.

And in my nervous and weakened condition most of such conversations, instead of being helpful and soothing, jangled my quivering nerves until I felt that I wanted to run or scream. I did not dare do either. If I did that the attendants and physicians forever after would set me down as insane in reality. All the patients already considered me as insane—else why was I locked up with them? And the attendants still were watching me, studying my every move to determine in what way I was not normal and why I should have been committed.

I found the gaze of one or the other of them on me frequently. I was a new patient. They did not know me yet. I must make no unconsidered move. I was compelled to keep to my chair, or go out on the exercising porch and walk monotonously back and forth, back and forth, back and forth.

If I sat in my chair for any length of time some patient was sure to come and seat himself beside me and start talking. Some of them could talk intelligently and seemed perfectly rational. But I soon found that these men flocked together and did not associate much with the other patients. Except while I was in bed these paid little attention to me. It was those whose minds were unquestionably warped who continually sat down beside me and forced conversation on me.

Even most of these men would talk rationally for a few minutes. Then suddenly their conversation would be quirked by their obsessions.

Their reasoning and judgment were twisted; they could not think in straight lines, their ideas and conclusions were grotesquely illogical. Yet I found quickly that if I did not agree with them they were apt to become either angry or disgusted with me. They could not realize that their ideas were fantastical or unsound.

They flung their obsessions and weird ideas at me almost continually. If I got up and escaped to the exercising porch they followed me, kept stride for stride with me and continued to talk. I could not shake them off or discourage them. I found that the patient who told me the "bugs would tie themselves on to" me if I paid any attention to them was eminently right. But his instructions were not complete. They failed to include detailed information on how to avoid paying attention to them.

And this constant drumming of distorted ideas against a person's brain is the most insidiously appalling thing that I yet have found about life in an insane asylum. Mental influences are not even given consideration in our present day handling of the insane.

Grimly I tried to set up a defense mechanism to save myself from the possibility of thinking along the irrational lines to which I was compelled to listen. I forced myself deliberately to study every man with whom I came in contact. And I learned volumes about the men who make up the great army of the locked-ins.

I found that some of them are perfectly sane. In fact a few of them are here strictly at their own volition—as a haven from what they consider a worse fate outside.

I am writing this in shame-faced apology. I, myself, permitted kindly intentioned friends to have me committed in order to cure me of a raving craving for liquor, a periodic craving on which I had spent thousands of dollars in private hospitals in an effort to secure release.

My friends finally concluded that only strictly guarded confinement over a long period of time could banish that blasting, recurrent, periodic craving. They had me declared insane—and I was too weak, physically and mentally, to fight against it.

To those scoffers outside who know nothing of deep-seated alcoholic addiction and believe that it requires only a conscious effort of the will for a cure, let me say that such a periodic craving is a recognized mental disease. Physicians call it dipsomania. It differs from the ordinary "whiskey thirst" as night does from day. It affects the mind, not only temporarily but sometimes permanently.

I wonder if I am as sane as I believe, or if, like the other patients, I can not realize my own aberrations.

But some of the insane have neither bad habits nor a scintilla of obsessions. Most of them may be divided into two general classes—those who have conspired to have themselves declared insane in order to escape trial or imprisonment on criminal charges, and those who are helpless victims of circumstances or the heartlessness of others.

This last class is not large but it exists. The men in the first class, those who have conspired to have themselves committed, are more numerous than the public suspects. But they get little sympathy or consideration from the hospital authorities. They are usually considered as criminal insane, are not given paroles, and the officials seem to bear down harder on them than on any others.

When I entered the hospital there were at least five men on the receiving ward alone who, by their own admissions or according to hospital records, had come here to "avoid the law." Their cases are typical.

One was a hardened youth, about twenty-one years of age, of the typical young gangster type. He was transferred to the hospital from one of the penitentiaries where he was serving a long term for felony.

He frankly admitted that he had "played crazy" for six months before his family and friends could get him transferred from the prison. He gloried in the fact that his "acting" had finally succeeded. He felt that he was more clever than the authorities of the penitentiary. But he did not immediately gain by the change.

In the hospital he was looked upon and treated as a dangerous criminal. He was locked in his room every night and never permitted to go outside the building, not even if accompanied by an attendant. Yet he was fully sane.

Political influence secured his release soon after I came to the hospital. A new governor was inaugurated and friends of the youth's father prevailed upon the new executive to give him a pardon from the criminal conviction. He was released from the hospital almost immediately; the superintendent knew he was not insane. But the patients here, who knew him, all laid verbal wagers that he would be back in a state prison before many months. He was just that kind.

Another one of the five got himself committed here to escape his responsibilities as the father of a nameless child. He had a wife and family so he chose to be declared insane rather than face court action on the part of the girl mother. I have never met the complaisant county judge who committed him. I do know his name. But I have the deepest contempt for him.

The story has spread around the ward. This inmate is held in contemptuous disdain by the other patients, even by those who are quite insane.

Still another of the quintet is a happy-go-lucky young man: an overgrown, playful boy; a fellow whose intentions are really good.

He had got to running with a wild crowd. The "bunch" had committed some depredation which ran it afoul of the law and this young man had assumed responsibility for the whole matter.

He came of a good family. He had numerous and strong friends. The authorities did not want to send him to prison for a long term but they believed he needed a good scare and a period behind locked doors. So they winked a sly eye when his friends, including his family physician, solemnly had him declared insane. He came to the hospital believing that a criminal charge had been filed against him in his home county. He learned later that the charge never had been filed, but that did not let him out of the asylum. He is still being held, so I suspect that the hospital authorities are not yet satisfied that he has had his lesson. Members of his family have attempted to secure his release but have not yet been successful. However I believe he will be released before very long.

Another man had an expensive family. In 1930 times became very hard and his over inflated business collapsed. But he and his family could not change their style of living. In a real estate deal he over-stepped the law. His attorney advised him to have himself declared insane. He accomplished it. But, like the rest of us, he does not know how long he will be here. That cuts deep on all of us; and he is becoming taciturn and gloomy. The charge against him has not been withdrawn. It may be waiting for him when he is released.

The class represented by these men does not include those persons of criminal tendencies more or less overlapped by obsessions or delusions. The latter are properly classed as criminal insane and should be sent to the asylum even before they commit a criminal act if their mental condition is known. They are a continual menace while at large.

But the men and women composing the second general class of the sane insane, those who are the victims of circumstances or the heartlessness of others, deserve the very deepest pity, in the majority of instances. It is not only sharply significant but a sad commentary on human inhumanity and present callous and archaic treatment of distress that a period of business depression, or hard times, brings these unfortunates to the asylums in greatly increased numbers.

Old people are brought in. So far as observation shows they are suffering from nothing more than the vagaries of the aged. Some of them are probably irritable, querulous or vacant minded. But all of us are familiar with such mental conditions in the very old. We do not consider them insane, but only in a natural dotage. Some show nothing more than a gentle childishness. Several of these have been received since I have been here. The attendants say, rather unemotionally, that the depression is to blame.

These old people can not earn a living. If they previously have been cared for by their families the members of the families may suddenly find that they are no longer able to stand the expense. Perhaps the breadwinner loses his job or is forced to less remunerative work. In the emergency he asks that the aged dependent be sent to the state hospital.

I believe that in many instances the person who applies for the commitment is misled by that euphonious designation, "state hospital." He visualizes a place where the aged will receive thoughtful, personal attention and kindly care.

No state hospital for the insane is a hospital in that sense. All of them are places for the confinement and guarding of large masses of insane; the discipline and methods of treating the inmates necessarily must be stern and harsh in order to fit the more uncontrollable patients.

Once committed here, the aged person must mingle with and associate with those really insane. He must follow rules of conduct laid down for the insane. Even in hospitals like this one, where an effort is made to segregate the harmless aged in special wards, the gentle, feeble old men must be congregated with some whose minds are badly warped, and attendants will still be guards, not kindly nurses. It is not a soothing contact and it is probable that the senile patients will not last long.

The year 1930 and the first month of 1931 brought a great increase in the number of persons committed to state hospitals, especially in those states most effected by drought, unemployment and general depression, hospital authorities say.

Very few of the additional cases admitted are due to insanity directly induced by the financial situation. A few such cases do occur. But those depressed by lack of employment or dire need are far more apt to seek relief through suicide than to become insane, official statistics prove. The increase comes largely from the cause above mentioned. But the dependents who thus are sent to the insane asylums include many who are not even aged. They may be physically deformed or even merely crippled to such an extent that they are unable earn a living. Such cases do come in, heartless as it may seem.

In a certain state there is no public hospital to care for indigent general-case patients. The counties have a poor fund and a poor farm. But during the fall of 1930 and the winter of 1930–31 numerous counties found their poor fund exhausted by necessary feeding of the unemployed and their families. There was nothing left to care for imbeciles and similar cases. So when families appealed to the county commissioners to take care of helpless dependents the commissioners took the easiest way—they applied to the county judge and he committed the unfortunates to the insane asylum.

This included victims of paralysis, mild epilepsy and harmless half-wittedness. Perhaps this is best, from one standpoint. The physicians at insane hospitals have had some experience in handling all kinds of mental cases and may be better qualified to care for such patients than the average county physician, who usually is strictly a political appointee.

There is another class of the sane insane. It is composed of persons suffering from malignant social diseases. Perhaps some city or county health inspector has discovered them working in a restaurant, butcher shop, bakery or dairy and has ordered their immediate discharge.

Shut off from the only occupation they know and without means to pay for private treatments, which are long drawn out and expensive if a cure is to be accomplished, they often take the most obvious way out. They manage to get committed to the hospital for the insane. Perhaps this also is best as this disease is rightly charged with causing several forms of insanity when not promptly and thoroughly arrested. A majority of these people probably would become insane later, and when the disease reaches that stage it is questionable if a full cure is humanly possible.

These are some of the facts which I gathered during that slow passage of time before I was called before the clinic. I gathered them from the patients, from the attendants, when I could manage to get them to talk to me for a few minutes, and from the ward physician. Getting information from the attendants was not easy. They are not there to give information to patients; they are there to control them. But the attendant in charge did unbend enough to give me a few facts after he had studied me for several days. I felt encouraged that he deigned to discuss any matter with me. Perhaps he did it in order to get a further insight into my mental make-up.

And my studied and unflagging prying after information had two good effects: it kept me from brooding on the lunacies of those around me, and kept me occupied while my body and mind were regaining strength.

However, in my study of the patients I quickly discarded the story which so many of them tell being "framed" and sent to the asylum by designing persons. In many instances they tell it that relatives or others "framed" them in order to get possession of their property, when they never owned a dollar's worth of property in their lives. In nearly every instance these tales are pure "moonshine," the physicians say. One of them had told me that in all the twenty years that he has been connected with hospitals for the insane he knows of but two cases where such a story was actually true.

But on this very ward, since that time, a case of "framing" was discovered which would challenge the attention of Believe-it-or-not Ripley. It is authenticated by the permanent records of this hospital.

The wife of a young farmer 'phoned county officers that her husband suddenly had gone hopelessly insane, and to come get him immediately as her life was in danger. The officers promptly arrested him and rushed him before the county lunacy board, which was composed of three general practitioners; physicians who knew nothing of insanity. Such boards often are so composed.

At the hearing that afternoon the wife described in minute detail how her husband had gone madly insane the night before, had suffered spells of wild, incomprehensible raving and repeatedly had threatened her life. The man denied the story completely but seemed to be puzzled and shocked by his wife's charges. The board hastily committed him and he was locked up on the receiving ward before nightfall.

The next day the wife went violently insane and was committed here on the complaint of several neighbors, supplemented by her own mad ravings during her hearing. Even the dunderheads on that smug lunacy board began to wonder if they had not made a mistake. A thorough examination of the man and his wife here brought out the fact that those physicians had committed a sane man on the complaint of an insane wife, and they had both man and woman before them at the husband's hearing.

The man was released and went back to his farm. Yet I wonder if his neighbors will believe his story or the one which the board members will devise to protect their professional reputations. The neighbors probably will believe the one the physicians tell, because they are doctors, while the farmer has once been committed to an insane asylum. Will not some suspicion of his sanity remain always in people's minds?

This, however, happened long after I had been examined at the clinic. From other patients I had heard about the clinic. Most of them pictured it as a sort of third degree in which the physicians ruthlessly pried into your past history, asked numerous highly personal questions, offered insinuations that you were not telling the truth, tried to trap you into damaging admissions and otherwise abused you.

So when the charge attendant, eight days after my arrival, notified me that I was to go to the office building that afternoon for a clinical examination I felt some quaking forebodings. But the clinic where I was examined was quite unlike the impressions given me.

One physician carried out the verbal examination. He was kindly and considerate. He put me at ease almost at once. Of course he went through the routine questions, asking me about any past insanity in my family and symptoms of insanity in myself, but he did it without offensiveness.

He inquired if I had any enemies who were troubling me, if I ever thought I heard voices singing, if I had visions, or if I had ever had periods of forgetfulness. I realized that he was studying my reactions to his questions far more than he was considering my answers. Almost before I knew it he had led me into telling my story in my own way.

I blurted out the full shame of it. I told him of the years and the small fortune which I had spent in my fruitless fight for release from my addiction. I told him of my final terrible debauch which had kept me lying in a private hospital, at death's door, for weeks, and how my friends had decided to have me locked up, regardless of the odium and the loneliness, in a last, desperate effort to cure me. I laid bare much of my pitiful self-analysis. And I knew that he was believing me.

Suddenly he turned to me with the question, "If I were to offer you a parole right now would you take it?"

God knows I wanted that parole. I wanted to get out into the air and the sunshine. I wanted to know that I could be trusted. But I had fought that question out with myself before I was committed to the hospital. I knew that when that maddening, periodic mental craving for liquor came on me I could not be trusted. I had proved that, time after time.

Even while I had been confined in a private hospital where I was paying out a tidy sum to be protected against my addiction I had bribed employees and secured whiskey. And I had done it while I was desperately swearing through clenched teeth that I would not yield to that awful demand of my brain.

So I told the doctor, very quietly, that I did not want a parole until I felt very sure that I was completely free of my craving. Till this day I am not sure whether the physician was really offering me a parole or whether he was testing my sincerity

But I do know that he took me at my word. I have never received a parole. I am still locked in,—and guarded.

Just as one of the patients had predicted, on that first day when I was permitted out of bed, things became far easier for me after my experience at the clinic. I am not sure whether the doctor had told the attendants about my case or whether they were beginning to realize that I could be trusted in most matters. I suspect that it was due to both causes. The doctor ordered me placed on a "special diet." In this institution that means that a patient may have one egg a day, and toast, a cup of milk, and soup occasionally, in addition to the regular menu.

Don't smile. Those scanty items make a wonderful addition to the usual fare. Eggs are never, at any time of the year, very obtrusive on the regular menu; and milk, for drinking, is almost unknown. Patients who have money deposited with the officials may buy milk and have it served with their meals but very few of them have the money.

But, better even than the improvement in diet, was the fact that I was given regular work to do. And work, to the asylum inmate, is an unmixed blessing.

My work was simple and easy; I was set at keeping a daily record of all important happenings on the ward, such as the admission of new patients, the hour of the doctor's and supervisor's visits, the packages received for the patients in the ward each day, with a record of transfers of patients to other wards or the infirmaries, and a record of all visitors.

I strongly suspect that the keeping of these records by a patient is not necessary. The attendants keep a separate record of the same occurrences. I believe the charge attendant gave me that work to do in order to occupy my mind and time and not because it is essential. But he deserves my thanks for putting me at it.

And how the better attendants do recognize that fact. One of the distinguishing marks of "good" attendants is that they are willing to spend time and thought in arranging to give each patient who can be trusted work suited to his ability. They lead him to believe that it is very important. The responsibility stirs him to do his best, and it also keeps him from brooding. Not all attendants are like that. Far too few of them are.

Many of the men are accustomed to outside labor before they are brought to the hospital. Shut inside, they are continually restless; irritably so. I have known of such men, who were too irrational to be trusted outside even under the supervision of an attendant, making a daily practice of begging the charge attendant, almost tearfully, to give them outside work.

Employment, during the summer, on the farm or in the greenhouse is considered a real privilege and the men strive to deserve to be given such work. On this ward the attendants dangle the greenhouse jobs as special prizes for good behavior.

But human nature inside an insane asylum is quite like that on the outside. A few of the men are willing to sit around and do nothing. The attendants have a very effective cure for that. Such men are almost invariably users of tobacco. The state supplies tobacco, of a sort, to the workers. If a man won't work he gets no tobacco. That usually brings them around. Almost any patient will work, and work well, until he earns a tobacco ration.

Tobacco is one of the greatest palliatives known for the loneliness of life on an insane ward. Let the reformers on the outside who would take tobacco away from the patients froth and rave about that.

I know that hospital attendants and physicians will fully agree with me in this, at least privately. Most of them do publicly.

If I had a friend in an insane asylum and did not send him tobacco and reading matter I would feel that the Sermon on the Mount had been wasted, so far as I was concerned; and the thirteenth chapter of I Corinthians could be considered a total loss.

By the time three weeks had passed my own path had been so smoothed by the physicians and attendants that it was far, far more bearable than at first. I had mind-saving employment, I had slightly better meals than many of the patients, I was permitted to come and go about the ward, and friends outside had sent me a little money which was kept for me by the officials and I could buy good tobacco. My home city morning newspaper had put me on its mailing list.

One friend, a woman, kept me supplied with magazines and other little comforts, in spite of my earnest efforts to persuade her not to do so. I appreciated the things; I hugged the mind occupation which they brought me. But I wished, and still do wish, that I could persuade or coerce her into forgetting me, completely and forever.

Her name, curiously, is Constance.

Our ward physician, who is also the assistant superintendent, had made out a room order for me without my asking him to do so, and when the first vacancy occurred I was assigned a room of my own. That was a wonderful relief. I no longer had to sleep in the dormitory with forty other patients. To some extent I could keep away from the fellows with the warped minds, and their distorted mental processes could not drum so constantly against my brain. There were a chair and a bureau in my room. I had some place to store my magazines and the few toilet articles which the woman friend at home had sent me.

While I was sleeping in the dormitory I had no place whatever in which to keep anything, except between the mattress and the springs of my bed, and then I had to keep a watchful eye on that bed all the time to keep some of the patients from surreptitiously appropriating anything they could find. And some of the cunningly sly ones could find the proverbial needle in a haystack—if they were forbidden to do so.

Yes, my lot was more bearable. But I was still locked in and guarded. The physicians saw to that even more thoroughly than I had expected when I had acknowledged that I was not to be trusted. The sunshine and fresh air of outside were not for a patient who could not be trusted.

I wonder just how long the road will be in my "beating back." I wonder just how long it will be before others can trust me; before I can trust myself. And I am legally insane. Will acquaintances and the world forget that? Or will my every thought and act be under constant suspicion, distorted in the minds of others by the fact that I have spent a time on the receiving ward? Can people, being what they are, merely human, be broad enough to understand?

And am I now, like the others, brooding, or am I bringing hard common sense to the solving of a real problem of my future? Am I competent to judge? I can not say.

Who can? No man knows the other man's mind, and no man can competently judge his own.

Prior to my being put through the mental clinic the physicians had had samples of my blood taken and tested. I had been vaccinated. My physical condition had been examined thoroughly. I learned that there was nothing of a serious nature organically wrong with me, although I was weak from long continued excesses. Time, rest and abstention from alcohol might overcome that. I need not worry greatly about my physical condition.

But I had never worried about that, so the knowledge was but slight relief. The things which keep me pondering moodily are quite different. Can that brain-ingrained periodic craving for alcohol be erased? Can I steel my mind to protect itself sufficiently against the constant wearing-down influence of distorted reasoning around me? Can that heavy mental torpidity, engendered by years of seeping my brain with liquor, be overcome?

But what troubles me more than any of these, as my brain slowly begins to think more clearly, is the question: Can I, having been one of the sane insane, face my thousands of acquaintances when I "go home?"

Have I "the guts to stand the gaff."

CHAPTER IV

LIGHTS AND SHADOWS

KIPLING once said, and it has been tremblingly repeated by other men, that "the female of the species is more deadly than the male." I am deeply convinced that Mr. Kipling, at some time, must have visited an insane asylum.

He was right—ask those who guard the insane.

We men patients are not permitted to associate with the women patients in any way, except under certain closely supervised conditions. Most of the time we can not even see them. Good, solid walls separate the sexes practically all of the time.

But if we can not see them we can very, very often hear them. And for my part I will be well pleased if I never hear another insane woman scream. My hunger for that sort of entertainment has been completely, and permanently, satiated.

This building is built in two wings; one occupied by men, the other by women. The wings are at least one hundred feet apart. The walls are thick and as nearly sound proof as sturdy construction will permit. Yet day after day and night after night we can hear wild screams issuing from the women's wing.

Often they are mindless, purposeless, unreadable screams, directed to no purpose and induced only by the hallucinations of a tortured mind. Such screams frequently excite other women patients and set them to screaming also, but their screams are shockingly different. They are made up of shameless profanities and disgusting obscenities. When the patients' screams are due to an acute paroxysm the women attendants try to soothe them. They administer mild sedatives, talk to them, cajole them. Sometimes, in extreme cases, they administer hypodermics.

But even hypodermics are seldom very effective in such cases.

An injection of morphine which would put a rational person into a sound slumber seems to have little effect on a paroxysm-driven mind. So far as I have been able to learn the patients are never gagged.

But if the screamer is actuated only by a perverse desire to scream she is given a very different treatment. If stern commands won't quiet her, and they seldom do, she is locked in her room and allowed to wear out her urge to scream. Sometimes she is put into a strait-jacket and tied to her bed.

But the screams come through the windows of the women's ward and dash against our windows, on this side of the open court. I have heard two or three of the patients in the women's wing of the building scream all night and through most of the succeeding day. And as I have tossed on my pillow, nerve-racked and sleepless from hearing those continuous, maniacal screams, I know that I could have mercilessly gagged the screamer, and suffered never a qualm of conscience. The women attendants have more patience than I have.

And the average person would be startled at the physical size and mental make-up of the women attendants. Very few in this institution are of more than the average height or weight. Some are slightly smaller than the average woman. Two or three are so small that it is a source of continual wonder to me that they are able to handle the women patients so efficiently. I do not know of one who is of the brawny, "fishwife" type.

They handle the patients largely through mental superiority, and a manner and tone of voice which I believe are acquired only through experience in handling the insane.

The men attendants of the better type acquire the same characteristics and tone of voice. It is surprising what effect these characteristics have on the men patients.

I have seen big, powerful insane men, in a fighting frenzy, brought to the hospital, shackled and handcuffed and guarded by two or more burly deputy sheriffs, and then seen a 150 pound attendant have the patient, with all bonds removed, under mental restraint and obedient to orders in a short time

Certainly it can not always be done. Force is sometimes very necessary. But often it is entirely needless.

But it is not only when they are in a paroxysm that the women patients are more troublesome, even more dangerous, than the men. Strip from any woman the inhibitions of heredity and constraint, and she is very apt to descend to depths or to go to lengths at which a man would balk with a sense of shame.

I know that the great army of women outside will make me rue that statement, if they ever get at me, after the state pulls its protecting wing from over my head. But just ask the physicians or attendants at an insane asylum. They know.

We are all familiar with what an intoxicated woman will do. Intoxication only lessens inhibitions. Insanity completely erases them.

I have seen a woman patient, at one of the dances here, raise a wild commotion and have to be forcibly removed from the floor in a fighting frenzy because a man patient with whom she had previously danced was dancing with another partner.

The hospital authorities here hold a dance for the attendants and the better patients, occasionally. The patients are permitted to dance only square dances but there are fox trots and waltzes for the attendants. The men patients behave in an orderly fashion; it is the women who require closest watching and sternest handling.

The hospital also has a film show for the patients every two weeks but the shows for the men and those for the women are not held on the same nights. The darkened room makes this impossible.

In telling me, the next morning, about the row the woman patient raised at the dance, a young attendant expressed the results of his experience. "No man patient would have raised a row like that in public, but the women,—well you can't tell what the women will do, except that it is apt to be something crazy. I can go up to any man patient on the floor and tell him to follow me and he will do it, but just try to tell one of these women to do something!"

Maybe I am wrong, but I believe that I can find a few reliable gentlemen who will admit that they have had some difficulty in inducing even a sane woman to do what they had told her to do.

It has always been my belief that women are, by inherent nature, more tidy than men. My experience here has sadly shaken that belief. I am wondering if their tidiness is not due to ideals instilled in them since birth, or to a desire to please others, especially men.

In one of the older buildings of this hospital the men and women patients formerly used the same dining room. The women came down to the dining room first, had their meals, and after they were returned to their wards the men came down for their meals. The plan was found impracticable because the women left the dining room so littered and untidy that the men could not stand it. The order was changed; the men ate first,—and kept the room sufficiently tidy and clean so that the women could use it afterward.

Now let the women fire their bombshells. If the barrage becomes too heavy I may be forced to tell just how constantly the women attendants have to keep spurring some of the women patients in order to get them to keep even their rooms and their persons clean.

Even among the insane there are characters which stand out; patients whose obsessions or bizarre quirks make them distinctive even in a general hodge-podge of quirks.

There is "Talking Louis." Louis holds no conversations with the rest of us; we are beneath his exalted and haughty notice. He talks only with kings and queens, and then only through an intermediary.

Just at present he is engaged in running the affairs of the whole civilized world through orders issued to members of the reigning British royalty. His imaginary intermediary is a young woman member of that family. He issues his orders to her and believes that she transmits them to the others.

He talks nearly constantly during the day and whispers most of the night. The day room may be very quiet when suddenly Louis' voice, commanding, stridently chastising, or mildly commending in tone, cracks the silence.

"I have previously told you that I can not be bothered by such small matters. Let the individual nations settle that. It is their problem. No! I tell you; and that settles it."

His conversations with his unseen *vis-à-vis* have no coherence, no continuing sequence; they are not connected with anything except his imaginings of the moment.

"What! Do you mean to tell me that boy is dead?" he suddenly burst out in anger, one afternoon. "I advised you more than a week ago that he was to be released, and you have let him lay there and die. No, I will accept no excuse. I made my decision and my wishes plain."

And a moment later: "Do you intend me to understand that he was in the city and did not call upon me?" Then his mind switched to an entirely different subject. "Yes he is a tenant of mine on my personal estate. He also rents two buildings from me in the city. He is reliable."

Talking Louis talks on; stridently shouting or importantly confidential by turns. If he becomes too strident the attendants stop him, but ordinarily they let him issue his commands just as he pleases. They have learned that nothing under the sun will entirely stop his talking. The other patients have learned to let him alone. Most of them seem never to hear him.

On the receiving ward, the "best ward in the institution," these unusual characters come and go. Sooner or later, in most instances, they are transferred to other wards. But a few manage to remain.

There is the man who is always right. No other opinion but his can possibly be reasonable. His church is the only possible door to Salvation; the others delude people to their damnation. His ideas of education are correct and all present schools are wrong, only leading young people into improper lives. An opinion contrary to his will set him almost frantic, and the man who expresses it is a hopeless fool.

I think I can hear someone saying that he knows men just like that who are not yet locked up. Quite true, except in degree. This man's bigotry has continually narrowed as he has been growing older, until it has become a mania.

Then there is Blondy, who is continually trying to escape. His mind is so far gone that his attempts are ludicrous, rather than dangerous. He makes a try at it every day or two, sometimes twice in one day.

Between the dining room and the kitchen the doors are kept open at meal times, and the kitchen has a door leading to the outside. Blondy has the impression that if he could just get into the kitchen he could get through that outside door, although it is kept locked. Also in the doorway between the kitchen and the dining room an attendant is always stationed during meal times, alertly watching everything that happens in the dining room.

Yet time and again Blondy will make a dash to get into the kitchen. He is always seized and dragged or chased back to his place at the table. But failures, even rather rough handling when he becomes threatening, never discourage him. Perhaps at the next meal be will try it again. Sometimes, instead of trying to dash past the attendant at the door between the two rooms he will undertake to force his way past. He will approach the attendant, his eyes blazing, his hands clenched into fists, his spindle legs tensed for the attack. In such cases the wily attendants just step to one side and as Blondy, thinking his way is clear, tries to rush by they grab him and drag him ingloriously back to his table.

Blondy, when seized, raises piercing shrieks, yells that he is being killed, and otherwise causes a hullabaloo, although I never have seen him get more than a scratch or two. He was formerly the manager of an important public utilities concern in one of the larger cities of the state, before his mind cracked.

Then there is the man who unceasingly carries a copy of the Bible. He hides it in his shirt whenever the attendants are around for fear they will take it from him. I have seen him, while waiting for the doctor to give him a hypodermic treatment for the malignant social disease which caused his mental breakdown, piously reading his Bible and marking nearly every other passage with a huge carpenters' pencil, his lips conning the passage devoutly. He is not kept on the receiving ward but I am told that he is sullen, unruly and wickedly profane in spite of his devout scriptural reading.

But it is Jimmy who would give visitors the greatest shock if he should happen to have one of his "spells" when any visitors were on the ward. Jimmy in a spell acts just like a cat in an old fashioned cat fit.

There seems to be no telling when he will "go blooie."

The other day he walked quietly into the day room. Then without warning be suddenly threw his arms around another patient and kissed him. The surprised and embarrassed patient pushed him away and Jimmy screamed, wild, horrifying screams. Then he turned and dashed into the dormitory, ran its full length and brought up with a crash against the farther wall, shrieking at every breath that he was "dying." He wheeled wildly, jumped upon a nearby bench and from it sprang so high into the air that he nearly touched the ceiling with his clutching fingers. He came down clawing at the walls with hands and feet. Then the other patients seized him. He clawed, screamed and fought as only a madman in a paroxysm can. But the moment he was placed in bed he became quiet and tractable. He did not have to be placed in a jacket or tied down. Most of the time he is docile, pleasant and apparently rational. Then he is off in another "spell."

Patients do not refer to such paroxysms as being crazy or insane. They say the suffering patient is "nervous," "disturbed" or has "a little spell." They are trying to soften their designation of his unhappy condition.

But, very inconsistently, the patients when discussing a man's ordinary condition will baldly refer to him as "crazy as a nightmare." Usually they do not let the man under discussion hear them unless he has angered them in some way. But if aroused they promptly tell the offending fellow patient that he is "crazy and always will be." Yet they respect his periods of paroxysms; perhaps because they realize their own aptitude to become "nervous."

But we have other quaint characters on the receiving ward. There is the "Concrete man." We all know him, and he lightens many hours for us as the other patients sit around and tease him about his queer obsession.

"I'm solid concrete inside, from my neck to my waist," he declares doggedly.

"Yessir, I am. You can't fool me; I know! I'm doomed to live for a thousand years. They won't let me die. Don't I know? I've tried it. Look there, —"

He displays his wrists, crossed with livid scars. His admission record is marked, "Suicidal," and when he was admitted to the hospital those scars were deep knife wounds, self inflicted. He had undertaken to prove that he was "doomed to live for a thousand years."

"There's no blood in me. I can't die. I cut those wrists and there was no blood." There was plenty of blood, but he believes he is telling the truth. "I'm solid concrete clear up to here?" He draws a bony finger around his neck. "I can't get nothing through me. I'm filled with concrete. I ain't eaten a bite or drank any water since I been here. What're you going to do when you're filled with concrete clear up to here?" Again he indicates his neck, while the other patients sit around and solemnly pump questions at him. After awhile he will tire of his tormentors and go off by himself, mumbling gloomily about being doomed to live for a thousand years, and will squat down on his heels with his back against the wall. He will squat there for hours and mumble.

He persists in claiming that he has not taken food or water since he was admitted although he eats a little at nearly every meal and drinks as often as most men. When relatives visited him recently he told them a harrowing story of how he had not taken food or water or had any bodily elimination for several weeks. I can not say how much of the story his visitors believed, but if they are like many other people who know only the life outside they probably believed there was much truth in it, and went away convinced that all the terrible things which most people believe, and seem to enjoy believing, about a "madhouse," are true.

My experience with "visitors" is that they come to a hospital to be shocked; they want to be shocked, and are disappointed if they are not.

As for yielding any of their ready-formed impressions about insane asylums and insane people,—wild broncos could not drag those creepy impressions from them.

The sane hug their delusions about the insane just as tightly, and a thousand times more fondly, than the insane hug their delusions about the sane. They enjoy creepy chills up the spine. Just where does sanity end and insanity begin, in this muddled world?

The man outside enjoys his delusions about the insane because he gets the same kind of crawly thrill out of them that an ignorantly superstitious person gets from chewing on his superstitions. If I am wrong time will tell.

In the same way that many Jews enjoy jokes told at the expense of the Jews, and many Scotchmen can appreciate a keen shot at the canny Scots, many of the patients, even some of those who are quite insane at times, like to hear or tell a good joke at the expense of their kind. Others may become violently angry at such jokes but I really believe they are in the minority.

Rough and ready jokes and good-natured horseplay arc common on the receiving ward, but even in these the patients must be careful who is the recipient. Even a friendly slap on the back may be misunderstood and violently resented by a patient who is having a "nervous spell."

The state, as represented by the hospital authorities, has recognized the fact that amusements may help and certainly can not retard a return of the patients to mental normalcy. There are a piano and radio receiving set in the day hall which patients may use, and those inmates who have musical tastes are permitted to bring their instruments to the hospital with them. Then for more general entertainment there are the winter dances, picture shows and Sunday religious services—which are a spiritual consolation for a very few and a welcome diversion for the majority of the patients.

Artistic tastes are seldom affected when minds go astray. In even the sadly insane artistic talents are generally retained. As one ward wit phrases it, "the reasoning may be bent but the artistic bent remains unbent." We have several good musicians on the ward, ranging from foot-patting fiddlers of hoe-down days to artists on the jazzy saxophone and 'cello. There are talented musicians in many of the wards. The orchestra which plays for the dances is made up almost entirely of patients, and don't think that the members can not play a snappy, late-model fox trot as well as they can render The Arkansas Traveler.

And those biweekly dances. Some of the patients are crazy about them, in ways that the lunacy commission never discovered when it committed them. Some of them, especially the women—excuse the dig—seem just to live for the next dance night.

They like them much better than the picture shows because the men and women can both attend the dances, while the two sexes must attend the film shows separately.

Not all of the unusual patients on the ward have quirks which amuse the others. The twisted personalities of many of them are distinctly unpleasant, even disgusting. There are not many of these on the receiving ward as they are transferred to other wards as soon as they develop such characteristics. But one or two remain.

There is Hilton, who does not have a well wisher on the ward. He is an epileptic but unlike many epileptics his mind is badly, and permanently, twisted; quirked into a mental nastiness.

He is highly disputative, sneering and gratuitously insulting. His very presence seems to be provocative. He can not carry on a short and casual conversation without making it replete with slurring remarks about either the listener or some other patient. The only reason that he frequently is not given a good beating by the other inmates is that any fighting is sternly repressed. When two patients get in a fight both are usually punished by being locked in their rooms or transferred to other ward, regardless of who is in the right. The fight also acts as a black mark against their record. So this man usually escapes, although a few of the patients have not been able to control their tempers and have given him what would have been a lesson if his mind had been able to reason out why he got the beating.

One insulted patient recently gave him a kick the groin which put him in bed for a week, but it had no effect on his nasty insultingness. He refuses to believe that his mind is not as sound as it once was; the other fellows get angry at what he says to them simply because "they are bugs."

Yet he is a skilled artist and musician, and his skill has not deserted him.

The walls of his room are covered with drawings and paintings which show a depth of conception and a deftness in execution which many excellent artists might envy, although all of his work evidences a trace of mysticism, a faint touch of the bizarre or weird. In an artist outside an asylum this bizarre touch would probably be accounted genius, but in a patient in such an institution it looked upon as a natural result of a deranged mentality so closely allied are genius and insanity.

There are shadows, sombre shadows, on the ward at times. There is, or rather there was, Little Barney. For Little Barney is not with us any longer. He died about a week ago in his bed in the dormitory, and I am afraid that brave Little Barney died in terrible torment. I know that he suffered, stoically suffered, excruciating agonies for hours before the end mercifully came.

Little Barney was only a boy not more than sixteen or seventeen years of age, small, emaciated, with his pitiful body twisted and distorted by the twin horrors of physical and mental diseases. He would lie in his bed, eyes wide with hallucinations and racking and suffering, but offering not a word of complaint. He might almost have been mute.

In the afternoon of his last day he developed a case of almost continuous vomiting. Before evening he was vomiting up blood, bile and mucus, and sympathizing patients said sadly, "Well poor Little Barney can not last long. He'll surely go tonight." About an hour before he died an attendant finally gave him some morphine in an effort to ease his pain, but it seemed to have little effect. His body was still writhing in agony when death wrenched his spirit free. But he died as he had lived—game. His lips never uttered a cry.

Perhaps not all of us recognized it at the time but Little Barney, with his patient suffering, was an inspiration to all of us.

He would lie there, racked body and soul by the agonies of his approaching end, but he kept his courage.

The Gray Wagon came for him. Next morning he was gone. There was grieving on the ward for him. We miss Little Barney.

It is not very often that the Gray Wagon, as some of the patients call the hearse, comes to the receiving ward. Few patients die on this ward, very few. The Gray Wagon stops more often at those wards which are designated as hospitals, because when patients become seriously ill they are usually hurried to one of the hospitals.

This institution has been established for many years, and men and women who came here fifteen or twenty years ago are reaching the end of their sad pilgrimage, every day or two. And the Gray Wagon must come for them. If they have no relatives or friends to claim their bodies they are laid to rest in the hospital cemetery.

But while death does not often invade the receiving ward it often sweeps close by. Recently a new patient was brought in. He was far gone with epilepsy. He should have been brought here sooner. During his first night he suffered about thirty convulsions. His body was scorchingly hot. Early the next morning the doctor came to see him. He took one look at the attendant's chart, another at the patient, now shaking in one of his almost continuous convulsions, and ordered him to the hospital. The patients who act as stretcher bearers came. The unconscious and spasmodically twitching man was taken to a hospital ward. He died just as they were placing him in bed. And just like the people who are still outside, we shook our heads and said, "He is better off."

Then there was one of our most trusted parole men. He was about fifty-five years old, white haired, rather distinguished looking and very intelligent. He was neat, pleasant, friendly and genuinely liked.

He worked at the hospital store. On a recent evening he left the store and started back to the ward. A few minutes later the attendants on the ward on the ground floor of this building heard something fall against the outer door. They opened it to find the patient's body slumped just outside. Heart failure had killed him almost instantly. And the Gray Wagon came for him.

There is a true story concerning his being here which heats my indignation to the boiling point; yet jolts my mind into pondering on the motives and qualities of character of Constance, the woman who refuses to forget me, even under my insistent urging.

He had been successful in business and had accumulated some valuable income-producing properties. His wife and he did not get along well; their married life was marked by frequent petty bickerings. When his reason cracked she had him confined in the state hospital, where his care cost her nothing. He apparently recovered. The authorities were willing to release him.

But his wife had discovered that the income he had built up, and into which she had come through having him legally committed, was sufficient to maintain her in comfort—and she was free of him so long as he remained locked up in the asylum. So she flatly refused to ask for his release, or even to permit him to be paroled to her. He was compelled to remain here.

So he died; admittedly recovered, but to all intents and purposes still insane; still one of the 300,000 souls in this nation who make up the great army of the Locked-Ins, who do not know when they are going home; whose terms have no set limits, for whom there can be but one of two ends:—recovery or death.

I wonder which door I will go through when I "go home."

CHAPTER V

Flying Feet

WHEN dance night comes there is a stirring around on every ward where any of the patients are fortunate enough to be permitted to attend. The attendants shave the men who are going, and there is a generous borrowing of clothing. I suspect the women emulate the men in this respect.

The patients, headed and flanked by attendants, are marched to the dance hall in double file. They are carefully counted and their names are taken down before they are permitted to leave their respective wards, and the attendants check them off every little while to see that none of them have "made a break."

At the auditorium, which is used for the dances, the men and women are seated on opposite sides of the room. Attendants to right of them, attendants to left of them, attendants in front of them, volley and thunder—at least they thunder—to keep the excited patients under decorum.

The dance numbers are alternated; a fox trot or waltz for the attendants and employees, a square dance for the patients. And it almost is worth a period on the receiving ward to witness one of these drag-and-haul affairs, from the vantage point of a patient.

When the square dance tunes ring out the men scarcely can be restrained. They must not rush across the room and choose partners until the supervisor gives the word. But when that word is given then the historic "run" into the Cherokee Strip of Oklahoma could have had nothing on the rush that ensues, so far as noise and confusion is concerned.

The women must remain seated until claimed, but they do not hesitate to signal a man, any man, and frantically, if they fear that they are about to be overlooked.

And how these attendants have learned to watch They are everywhere; women as well as men.

They have their hands full, watching the dancers, getting them properly started, coaching them to follow the calls, guiding them through the figures where necessary, seeing that no couple dances out of turn or out of place and sternly curbing any incipient disturbance.

This latter is abundantly needful. A dance, even among the "cultured circles" of our cities, is apt to generate some jealousies; among people whose judgment and repressive faculties are loosened or unhinged it is far more certain to do so.

Of course only the better patients are permitted to attend the dances but among the five hundred men and women who usually crowd the hall there are certain to be some who may cause a disturbance if not kept under strict discipline.

No introductions are necessary. The men simply select the women with whom they want to dance and the women never decline. A few sometimes evince an exaggerated coyness which gives the spectators a hearty chuckle, but usually the women are so anxious not to be overlooked that they jump at the first man who signals them by an airy wave of his hand.

And the dances! What a hub-bub and burly-burly they are! There is no regular number of couples to a set; just whatever number crowds in. The set ends when the supervisor blows a shrill whistle, and he tries to see that each couple has a part in going through the figures of the call. The men leave the floor decorously when the music ends. There is little masculine "showing off." The women sometimes linger on the floor until ordered to their seats. Sometimes one or two must be removed forcibly.

The women are permitted to dance round dances with other women as partners, but only a few avail themselves of the privilege. What they come for is to dance with men. However, there are some beautifully graceful dancers among the women patients.

The music seems to permeate them, to control them. They are a part of it, dancing to its rhythm in perfect consonance, discarding stereotyped and mechanized steps, expressing each beat and accent by responsive movements of their bodies.

How some of our mechanical-minded 'interpretative" dancers would be improved if they could only become temporarily insane when entertaining a group of tired business men!

There is one girl, clear-eyed, vivacious, apparently fully sane, who draws my eyes whenever she gets on the floor. What a dancer! Swinging around in the arms of some other girl, but nevertheless vibrantly expressive of the music. How I would enjoy a waltz with her! But that is not for me. I am a patient—and that is that.

And such a commingling of party dresses, the plain print dresses supplied by the state, and the white uniforms of the women attendants! And what a medley of civilian clothing, shapeless state suits and even overalls as the men flaunt! It is a complete democracy; about the only one remaining in this world of "front" and pretense. Others are hollow pings of democracy's forms and trappings without achieving a democratic mind. This is a democracy of mind; social planes and mental reservations all have been swept away.

Not that most of the women and many of the men do not do their poor best at decking out for the occasion. They do that with a vim—in order to make a good appearance before the other sex, and not to indicate social standing. There is no social standing at these dances. Former standing is completely ignored and unconsidered. You may have been a charwoman, a waitress or a debutante; a hobo, a dairy hand or business executive on outside; but here you are just one of the patients, hungering for physical expression and association with the opposite sex. And that is back to first principles, in sincerity.

Oh, yes; smug ladies and gentlemen—those are the things which did, and to an unacknowledged extent still do, motivate the human race. Scratch off your own superimposed civilization and refinement and see what you find.

That is, do it if you are broadminded enough and self-honest enough to admit what you do find. If not, then why not join us here.

Smile that pityingly superior smile, darn it; and go back to your luncheon clubs and bridge teas.

But I have wandered clear away from the dances, and the vivacious girl who dances what the music tells her to dance. She always wears a red party dress. And, yes she uses some lipstick. So do all the others who can get it. And if I were a woman and had a relative or friend in a hospital for the insane and did not send her a lipstick I would not feel qualified to attend church the next Sunday; certainly not to take Communion. And I might include a carton of cigarettes with the lipstick, if the lady was addicted to them before she was locked in.

The women attendants would promptly confiscate the cigarettes, but my conscience would be as clean as a baby's.

Heigho! My teasing mind just won't behave. Somehow the thoughts of the girl in the red party dress, and other women patients who are rational along most lines of thought and at most times have set me to philosophizing.

And that is exactly the effect that the dances seem to have on some of the other patients. Attempts at escape can sometimes be traced to the limited association which the men have with the women on dance nights.

The patients get to thinking of the outside, and of the things of which they are deprived while being held in the asylum. An overpowering revolt against their fate surges up within them.

In the parlance of the locked-ins they suffer from "stir fever." Then they plan or attempt an escape.

Only one attempt in ten succeeds even temporarily, and only about one in fifty results in freedom for any considerable time. This is not because some of the patients are not capable of startling cunning in planning escapes, but because that cunning is nearly always offset by ludicrous blundering due to lack of clear reasoning ability.

There is another factor militating against a successful escape by an insane patient. It is the fact that he can so easily be apprehended by peace officers, even the most unskilled. A country constable or the town marshal of a Main Street village can recognize a person who is badly insane, especially if he is suffering from unusual excitement, as an escaping patient always is.

Then very, very few patients, except some of the parole men, have any money. If they are successful in getting away from the hospital they have no place to go except back to their homes, where their condition is known. If they go there the members of their family are afraid of them, in most cases, and won't harbor them. The hospital authorities are generally notified of their whereabouts by members of the family or by some neighbor who is in physical fear of having the patient loose in the vicinity.

Without money or suitable clothing and with the hospital pallor on their faces, even those patients who are rational most of the time and have no appearance of being insane, have but little chance of getting employment, and some of those who have escaped and tried for days to get work have crept back to the hospital doors and given themselves up in order to get something to eat. They are starved into coming back.

No sirens shriek when a patient in an insane asylum escapes from the grounds. There is no ringing of bells and the other busy hubbub which follows the escape of a convict from the penitentiary. The hospital authorities simply notify the peace officers of the county from which the patient came and the local police department, then wait until the patient is brought back. Usually he is back within a few days, and after that he is watched so closely that he has little opportunity to repeat the "break."

There are no wholesale attempts at breaking out of an insane asylum. The mental condition of insane patients seems to preclude entirely their cooperating in escape attempts. They act alone. They keep their plans, if they are able to plan, entirely to themselves. They do not act in concert in anything; they are completely individualistic.

Escapes are attempted so often that they become commonplace to the officials. Patients who realize that they are insane know that they are locked up for life unless they recover. Those who are convinced that they are not insane usually realize that the physicians are not so convinced and will continue to hold them. Hence, since nothing which they may do can increase the length of time for which they are locked up, they feel that they have little to lose by trying to escape. Brooding on this, they try it.

In doing so they furnish a welcome break in the dead monotony of the other patients, who have something exciting to talk about for several days. And how they will chatter about the break when the attendants are out of earshot. They are quick to spot the blunders of the man who has tried to get away. "Now he was a fool to try it that way," one of them will say. "If it was me I would have —" He will outline the plan he would have used, which usually is just as full of holes as was the unsuccessful one.

They always hear of any escape or anything else of importance which happens in the institution. The "grapevine" works rather efficiently even in an insane asylum, though, of course, it is not developed to as high a degree as it is in prisons where the inmates are all sane, or are classed and handled as such.

I have never ceased to wonder at the remarkable way that news spreads in this institution. I have learned of escapes from some other ward before the attendants on this ward have learned of them. I have learned details of a violent spell of a patient on another ward when I was totally unable to puzzle out any means of communication between the patients of the two wards.

Some patient would whisper the news. We never ask how it is gleaned. I always hesitate to believe stories brought to me in this way until they are verified. Like all rumors they may be badly distorted by repetition. Then many patients are prone to great exaggeration or are mentally incapable of drawing reasonable conclusions. But stories brought to me by "grapevine" usually have sound basis in fact even when distorted in the telling.

It is the men holding grounds paroles who are most often able to reach home before being apprehended, following an escape. They are mentally better able to plan, have far more opportunities than the others, some of them have a little pocket money, and most of them do not appear insane.

An almost positive proof that insane men are in some manner psychic or develop an ability to guess what the other man is thinking is given by the fact that other patients nearly always guess when a man is planning an escape. Sometimes the effort is frustrated by some patient telling an attendant of his suspicions.

Other patients knew that one of the parole men on this ward was planning to escape several days before he made his successful effort, yet he had told his plans to no one.

Attendants advance the theory that the patients noticed that this man was quiet and brooding and jumped to the true conclusion. I think not, but at any rate they guessed right.

The unparoled patients, who are kept locked in, have only the very slimmest chance to escape. The wards are so arranged and handled that the attendants have the patients under watch at all times. Then most of them are unable to plan coherently.

Recently the attendant in charge of this ward had a number of the patients cleaning a new building which had just been completed by the contractors and had not been occupied. No matter in what room the patients were working the doors were kept locked. But the attendant finally stepped into another room for a moment leaving the door unlocked but setting a parole man beside it with orders to see that no one got out.

The attendant had scarcely left the room until one of the patients, a full-blooded Indian, went to the parole man and told him that the attendant had given him permission to go for a drink of water. The parole man believed him and permitted him to pass through the door. He made his way outside before the attendant returned to the room.

Of course the attendant missed the Indian immediately and dashed out doors looking for him. Before leaving the room the patient had not stopped to think that getting out of the building was not all that was necessary, as he would still be within the grounds.

But once outside the building he realized that he must not run as that would attract attention, so he undertook to walk unconcernedly to the boundary fence. This gave the attendant time to sight him and the Indian was caught at once. He gave up without remonstrance but was transferred to other and stricter ward for the attempt. He will be closely guarded in the future.

Men who have had penitentiary "training" before being brought to the hospital sometimes give trouble by attempted escapes. One such man recently persuaded a boy patient to purloin a file from the art department in which the boy worked during the day. He hid the file in his shoe until he had an opportunity to use it. So far the ex-convict had planned like a sane man. His next step was characteristically that of an insane patient.

He undertook to file the lock which secured the hinged frame of bars which covered the window in the ward lavatory. Since someone is almost continually going into or coming out of the lavatory at all hours, day and night, the attempt was discovered and the patient was transferred to the ward where the criminal insane are kept, while his boy accomplice was denied the privilege of working in the art department.

In this department baskets, rugs, toys and bric-a-brac are made. The work is light and pleasant and relieves monotony, so it is considered a privilege to work there.

Relatives who visit patients sometimes unwittingly stir them up to try to escape. They bring all the news from home. They try to cheer the patient by telling what good times they had on a party, a fishing trip or a visit to the theater. Such things are maddening to a man shut off from all such enjoyment. The very solicitousness of some visitors reminds the patient of the repression and discipline of the ward. The visitors, feeling that they have done the patient a "world of good" go away and leave him brooding on the barrenness of his own life, and he may attempt an escape.

But there are a few cases where relatives actually incite the patient to attempt to escape, or abet his efforts to do so.

The father and mother of a young man patient visited him here not long ago. They persuaded one of the physicians to accompany them and the boy out on the grounds—to give the boy some air. As soon as they were outside the building the mother produced two pocket knives from her handbag, handed one to the boy, kept one herself, and the three of them attempted to bluff their way out of the grounds by threatening the physician with the knives. The physician managed to argue with them until attendants could come to his assistance.

Mother, father and son had to be overcome by force. Yet the boy was undeniably insane and belonged in an insane asylum. Really I believe his mother belonged here also. I am quite sure that his father did, for permitting his wife to persuade him to join in the foolish attempt. He laid all the blame on her shoulders.

Let's think; didn't Adam do something like that when the Lord asked him who ate the apple? But I have been told that they did not have insane asylums then, so they just committed Adam to the custody of his wife—for life. I wonder if that is not really what made him sweat.

Letting Adam lie, however, and getting back to the hospital, the patient who makes a wild dash while lines of patients are being marched from one building to another has practically no hope of gaining freedom. Life in an insane asylum, without regular exercise, soon deteriorates the muscles, the patient is seldom in condition to run fast or far, and an attendant soon overhauls him. This is true even at night as the grounds are brilliantly lighted. The runner has little chance.

At least that is what those of us who consider ourselves sane believe—but wait a minute. I have to admit, sheepishly, that most of us consider ourselves sane. So there.

But one young man here beat the unbeatable by making a sudden dash while the patients were being taken to a dance.

He got clear away, reached home, then typed a genially chaffing letter to the charge attendant, giving all the details of his escape. He was a young married man and his wife had had him committed to cure him of a violent jealousy. With the names changed, his letter read:

"Dear Mr. Oglethorpe: I 'sorter' hated to treat you like that, but thought maybe the gang would get more of a kick out of seeing a speed demonstration than they would out of a musical recital. Guess it would have been more exciting if some one besides that big, fat attendant had chased me. Sure was some yelling he did.

"When I looked back at the fence and saw no one pursuing, it was a mighty grand and glorious feeling. That first field I went through was terrible. I sank nearly to my knees in mud, water and snow, and for the first half mile it was a mighty struggle. I had eaten a big supper and was in no condition for rapid progress.

"I ran east until I got into the timber, turned southwest toward the railroad tracks and ran about three miles before I reached them.

"Never dreamed there were so many fences in the whole state. I got into one vineyard, or something, which had a chicken-wire fence every ten feet or so for a quarter of a mile, it seemed. I struck one creek but finally found a foot-log. As it was so very dark I got down on my hands and knees and 'cooned' it.

"Then I walked right on down the railroad tracks. When I reached Advent my limbs had got so stiff they would hardly bend and in order to move one of them I simply had to sling it sidewise. At Advent I climbed into a box car on a siding to lie down and rest a bit, but soon became so chilled by the cold that I crawled out and crippled on down the track. And say, but that night was a long one.

"Finally I heard some roosters crowing for day, and about that time I saw a light come on in a farm house away over from the tracks and I headed for it. The old lady came to the door, and when I told her I had walked all night and would like to come in and get warm she said it was only about twenty minutes to five o'clock and that she was not getting up, but was only seeing what was wrong with the dog. Seemed he had become uncomfortable in some way; he was sleeping in the bed with them.

"The old man rolled out and invited me in; then built a fire in the cook stove and I had the goodest breakfast ever. Oatmeal, eggs, hot biscuits and honey. About sun-up I started creeping down the highway, badly hampered in my stride, and very painful, here and there.

"Several cars passed me up, but finally, one stopped; a big sedan with the president of a utilities company in it. When I asked him where he was going and he said Martinsville I decided the Good Lord was right with me. It meant he would drop me just two blocks from home. I got here in time to help wash the breakfast dishes.

"It is a glorious feeling to be at home, but I am proud that Mrs. R—— sent me up there. It jarred me out of a trend of thought that was making life unpleasant for us all, around here. And I will always feel grateful to you, Mr. Grimes, et al, for your kindly consideration.

"Please open the little Christmas box Mrs. R—— sent me and return the two $1 bills therein and the handkerchiefs. Then you and Mr. Grimes cabbage on to the fruit cake. Mrs. R says she used a little something besides water to mix it up with, and that if you happen to be a bone dry you may not like it.

"Mrs. R—— wrote to Superintendent Addings today to mail my clothes, dictionary, keys, etc. to her. Sorry to put you to that trouble."

"Merry Christmas to you and yours, and a happy New Years.

M.L.R.

P.S. We are getting ready to drive down to the farm and I wrote this in a hurry. 'Spect' I hit some wrong keys, and didn't spell much 'good.' I still believe that it is possible for some good to come out of anything—even the activities of a bedbug. And I realize that much good has come from my visit with 'you all.'" M. L. R.

The "court of final appeal" in here, which consists of all of us who are in on a bit of news, has studied the case of M. L. R. and has handed in a verdict. It reads, "If that sort of man was jealous his wife probably gave him good cause to be."

I believe that the hospital authorities agree with the opinion of the "court." Certainly I have learned of no strenuous efforts to bring M. L. R. back.

CHAPTER VI

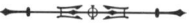

BARS AND STRONG ARMS

SPRING has come; the trees outside are breaking into leaf; the grass is green and inviting; everything is stirring, growing.

Business men, in the world outside, idling at their desks, are dreaming of seed catalogues and garden spots, with the smell of newly turned earth; or of golf courses, and fishing streams. And the men who are locked in are restless, stirring, morose and uneasy.

The urge of spring affects the men on insane hospital wards far more noticeably, and poignantly, than it stirs their freer fellow men. If you are chained to your desk in the spring time your work becomes positively galling, although there is time after office hours to play nine holes and work up a satisfying perspiration, or even to try out your car along roads bordered with green. If you are a boy in school your willful mind constantly flits to the great outdoors, although there are recess times and a couple of hours after dismissal. But if you are locked in an insane asylum, tramping back and forth on its hard, bare floors, spring restlessness produces sullenness, irritability and hair-trigger tempers, And among men whose mental poise is precarious this leads to quarrels and fights.

There is physical violence, at times, on any ward of any hospital for the insane. This is not only according to my experience here; attendants, long experienced in many hospitals, tell me that this is true. Most of them add that there always will be violence in asylums as long as insanity exists.

Insane patients inevitably will develop sudden and unpreventable fights among themselves or become violent and have to he restrained by force. Some of them will attack or defy attendants; and attendants, being human, sometimes will use stern force when it is neither necessary nor just, much as some school teachers sometimes administer a whipping when other methods would be better.

But there is very little unjust violence toward the patients in this ward and I am told that it is much the same throughout the institution. Any "rough stuff" which becomes known brings a quick investigation on the part of the hospital authorities.

And necessary physical restraint of patients must not be confused with brutality. They are in no wise synonymous.

I have seen plenty of physical clashes, even on the receiving ward, since I have been here. I have seen numerous bloody noses and battered faces, but I have seen only two instances where an attendant deliberately attacked a patient and I have never seen a patient injured by an attendant beyond a few scratches and ordinary bruises.

The attendants know just how to take hold of patients to render them helpless and subdue them. They are trained in a sort of elementary jiu-jitsu, and long experience teaches them to outthink the patient in a physical clash. Some of them do lose their tempers or their heads and handle patients brutally or unjustly, but only seldom. On the other hand attendants are more often attacked by patients in an insane paroxysm or an unreasoning rage.

The ward was still, at 3 o'clock the other morning. Patients were sleeping peacefully. Suddenly there was a wild commotion in the day hall, followed by the thud of a falling body. I sprang out of bed and rushed for the day hall. So did numbers of other patients. I had acted quickly, but two other patients were before me. When I dashed into the day hall they had seized a struggling patient and thrown him to the floor. The night attendant, with blood streaming from his nose, was just picking himself up off the floor, ten feet from where he had been sitting a few minutes before.

He never laid a hand on the violent patient. Other patients attended to that. They had him stretched out on the floor and helpless in a jiffy. The attendant brought a strait-jacket but it was the other patients who put it on the violent one, carried him to his bed and tied him down, with the attendant, of course, supervising the work.

Then the facts came out. This particular patient was one who had always appeared quiet and tractable. The attendant was seated at his table when the patient came out of the dormitory, apparently headed for the lavatory. Just as he passed the table he wheeled on the attendant. "Give me those keys," he shouted. As the attendant started to rise from his chair the patient crashed out his fist with frenzied strength, knocking the attendant out of his chair and to the floor.

The attendant was wearing an eyeshade and so fierce was the blow that he was literally knocked from under it: the eye shade falling to the floor several feet from where the attendant landed. There was reason for the blood that the attendant dripped all over the floor while the man was being placed in the jacket; his nose was broken. Yet the next morning the patient was released from the strait-jacket and went about his duties as usual. The only punishment he received was to be transferred to another ward.

One afternoon a strongly built but very quiet new patient was being checked in and bathed. One of the older patients was assisting in bathing him. Suddenly the new patient sprang erect and smashed a wicked right-hand blow to the mouth and nose of the older patient. The blood fairly streamed. There was a mad scramble for a moment or two, then one attendant and the older patient had the new man down and helpless.

The attendant used a hold which is a favorite one with attendants when a patient becomes violent. In asylum parlance it is known as "Necking."

He seized the fighting man from behind, threw his left arm around the patient's neck with his forearm pressing upward against the chin and his right hand locked around his own left wrist. The hold is very like the strangle hold in wrestling but is applied from behind. The patient finds the grip like a vise, and since his back is toward the attendant he is helpless to do much return damage. The attendant simply maintains his hold until the patient exhausts himself by his struggles, or till other attendants or patients seize and overpower the frenzied man.

In neither of these two cases did the attendants strike a blow nor did the attacking patients later receive any physical punishment or mistreatment whatever. Both of those attendants happened to be "good" attendants.

Tales drift to me via "grapevine" of men being abused in other wards, and some of the patients on this ward have told me of being knocked down and abused unjustly on other wards or in other hospitals. It is difficult to know just how far to believe these stories. A man in a paroxysm or even a rage is not capable of judging his own acts or those of others.

This can be almost as well applied to the majority of men outside. I have not found many sane men who would acknowledge that they were in the wrong after a fight. The other fellow is always in the wrong.

I can get a pretty accurate idea of what took place in a clash here through the opinions of disinterested insane patients who saw the trouble. If they generally agree that the patient "got only what he deserved" I am quite sure the attendant was not to blame. The majority of patients are accurate in their judgment of the justice or injustice of the treatment of others than themselves.

A story sifted like wild fire through the hospital, a week ago, of how a patient had been choked to death by an attendant and several patients who were trying to force a dose of salts down his throat.

It happened on another ward, so I do not know the exact truth of the matter. But some of the parole patients tell the story another way. They say the patient suffered from a weak heart; that he was not hurt in the least during the struggle, but that after he was released his heart failed to stand the exertion and excitement and he died, in bed. My guess is that this is the correct version. I know that many patients refuse to take medicine, or even to bathe, when ordered to do so. They must be forced to do as ordered, as no attendant can maintain his ascendancy over the other patients if he permits one to defy him.

One of the patients here tells me a story which illustrates what some of the patients think of an attendant who lets the patients disobey him. And judging by the opinions of some of my associates here I can well believe the story, although its events took place in another hospital.

"There was a new attendant on the ward where I was then," the patient says. "He did not know how to make some of these nuts behave. He told a fellow to go sit down and the fellow would not do it. Then one of the other patients just whaled away and knocked the stubborn patient down and jumped on him and bumped his head on the floor. When they pulled him off and asked him why he did it he said he was just showing that 'nut' they had up there, trying to run the ward, how it should be done."

Patients often side with the attendants in any difficulty with other patients, if they see it and believe the attendants are in the right. But they never forget a brutal act; they remember it and talk bitterly about it, yet practically no attacks on attendants are the result of grudges—the insane mind does not seem to work that way. Those most insane seem to act only on sudden impulses. The only ones who retain dangerous grudges are those most nearly sane. The patients are bitter against brutal attendants but do not translate that bitterness into acts. Perhaps they are afraid to do so.

Unconsciously and unadmittedly the really insane realize that they are in some way inferior to the sane; they fear the attendants far more from a mental than a physical stand-point. Very few of them will even complain to the physicians when they have been the victims of mistreatment. They give various excuses for not doing so.

"What's the use?" one patient said to me. "They won't believe me. They'll believe the attendant. They think I'm just a damned insane man. Then if I complained the other attendants would just make it harder on me."

There is some truth in that, but the real reason this man does not complain is that he has an indefinable fear of the mental ascendancy of the attendants. But the physicians sometimes learn of attacks on patients without the injured patient complaining.

One patient, now on this ward, went to the aid of an attendant who was having a fierce fight with another patient. The attendant was either too angry or too excited to know that this patient was trying to help him and he knocked his would-be helper down, jumped on him and repeatedly bumped his head on the concrete floor. The patient received some bad contusions, but he did not complain to the physicians. However, the ward physician noticed the contusions. He asked the attendant how the injuries had been incurred and the attendant answered flippantly that he supposed the patient "had been kicked by a mule." That flippancy was a mistake; an investigation followed and the attendant was discharged.

Visitors, those actuated by morbid curiosity—and how I hate to see them come—usually ask to see "the cell rooms." They want to be shocked. Patients tell me that cell rooms do still exist in some older hospitals but there is not a cell room, of the kind usually visioned, in this institution. The rooms in which the criminal insane are confined are exactly like the one in which I am sitting as I write.

They are small rooms, about eight by ten feet in area. The thick walls are of concrete, smoothed and painted. Even the door is smooth. There is no knob, inside or out. There are a strong lock and a handle on the outside of the door but both are set flush with the surface of the heavy oak door so that patients may not bump against them.

The windows are double barred. In addition to the heavy bars which are let into the brickwork of the window frame there is a steel frame of far lighter bars so closely placed that it would be very difficult for anyone outside to pass a weapon between them. This frame is hinged on one side and secured by a padlock on the other. This is to allow of these frames being opened when it is necessary to wash the windows. But the heavy bars can not be moved and we, —yes, we, —must wash the windows by reaching between them.

The difference between the criminal and violent wards and the one in which I am confined is that of stricter discipline, closer supervision, fewer privileges, sterner attendants and continual association with criminal insane.

On every ward painstaking care is given to seeing that nothing which might be used as a weapon is to be found. Even on the most violent wards the attendants carry no weapons. It would be the height of folly to permit them to do so. With two, or at most three, attendants locked in a ward with fifty or sixty insane men there is too great a possibility that some of the patients would wrest away any weapon which an attendant might have. In a clash between patients and the men set over them it is a battle of natural weapons; of muscles and wits.

Even in the dining room great care is taken. Not only are the knives, forks and spoons collected and counted at the close of each meal, but heavy pitchers are taboo. In another asylum in this state a heavy, glass syrup pitcher, filled with syrup, was set on one table.

A patient discovered its weight just as an attendant passed the table. He sprang to his feet and crashed the glass pitcher against the attendant's temple, with all the power of a frenzied arm. The attendant dropped in a heap to the floor, his skull fractured. He died the next morning.

On "shave days" extra care is taken. All patients on a ward are shaved by the attendants, and every attendant must be at least a passable barber to be qualified for his job. He must know, also, that he can not lay his razor down for even a moment. One shave day, here, an attendant on this ward slipped his razor into the outside pocket of his jacket for a moment. A "suicidal" patient saw the act. Stealthily he filched the razor, dashed into the dormitory and cut his throat from ear to ear, before the attendants could reach him. He died gloating that he had been able to carry out his purpose. And the Gray Wagon had to make another trip.

The nozzles of the fire hose, coiled high on racks in the hall, are riveted on. Trust some patient to find it out if they could be screwed off; and a twelve inch bronze nozzle would make a wicked weapon in the hands of an insane man. The steam radiators are slung from the ceiling, high up out of reach and where no patient in a fit might fall against them.

I have yet to see a pair of shackles or handcuffs here. I am told that they have them for use in transporting patients to other hospitals, but I have not found a man in the institution on whom they have been used, after arrival here. Several patients have told me, however, that they knew of patients being shackled in other institutions where they were previously confined, and I have seen patients brought to this hospital, by officers, handcuffed, shackled or both. Peace officers are far more afraid of the insane than are experienced attendants.

They are just like the balance of mankind; they are afraid of anything which they do not understand. We are afraid of death because we do not understand it. So we accept, invent or conjure up religions as a partial palliative for the terrors of the unknown.

Some fellow, whom I am confident had never been a patient in an insane asylum, once wrote that iron bars do not make a prison—or words to that effect. Well, maybe so! But how those iron bars can remind you of a prison, if you happen to be on the locked-in side of them. And there are many other things which constantly remind me of where I am.

There is a tiny, square opening in the door of my room at a height level with a man's eyes. It is there to permit the attendants to look into the room before opening the door. Often it is the better part of valor to look through the small opening and see where the patient is, what he is doing and what he may be intending to do, before unlocking the door.

A patient in a spell often is prone to come through the doorway fighting, the minute the door is unlocked. And the door to my room has such an opening, just like the rest. Then every time I go down to the dining room I am reminded. Attendants must unlock the doors, watch us narrowly while we eat, marshal us back upstairs and lock the door behind us.

I am reminded every time I look at my finger nails. I clean them with a toothpick and pare them with a nail clip, borrowed from an attendant. And I used to get a manicure with every second shave; here I did not even have the toothpicks to clean them with until Constance, on a visit to me which I had vainly forbidden her to make, caught me picking my teeth with a straw which I had salvaged from a discarded broom.

Write down "toothpicks" in your list of what the well equipped insane patient should have.

Those two boxes of toothpicks which Constance sent me enabled the boys who like to play cards to have a poker game in the card room—when the attendants are not around. Prior to that they had nothing to use for chips. The toothpicks are not fully satisfactory as poker chips, however. Some of the fellows are forever wanting to borrow a part of your stack to use in cleaning their pipes.

There are other reminders of where I am. I am reminded whenever Constance comes to visit me. To reach my room she has to pass through the day hall, with all the patients peering at her; eyeing her furtively, suspiciously, leeringly, or acquisitively, according to their differing natures.

I am reminded when she tells me about affairs in my home city. Other men are filling the places which I used to consider mine; are heading community fund drives, sitting in my seat on civic committees, filling the editorial space which formerly was kept sacred for what I had to say; are forging ahead—keeping in the public eye. And I—I am polishing floors, wielding an inept broom, awkwardly making my bed, and skinning my knuckles as I reach between the iron bars to wash the window of my room.

I am reminded by the shrieks which daily and nightly come from the women's ward across the court. I am reminded by the 8 o'clock call of "Bed time." I am reminded by the bickerings and the fights among the patients on my own ward. I am reminded by the necessity for my unflagging efforts to close the doors of my mind against the insidious effects of the distorted ideas of those around me.

I am reminded—more than by anything else, I am reminded—by every new batch of thrill-hungry visitors which comes on the ward. My hackles rise whenever the attendant shouts, "Visitors on the Ward," just before they are admitted.

They peer at me, baldly ogle me. They stare in my door with gaping-mouthed wonder when they see me pounding my typewriter. They wonder what my obsessions are, and whether I am hallucination-driven and so must be forever and forever punching so viciously at the keys.

Figuratively they are licking their lips as they peer at the curiosity before them.

And they don't seem to realize that I am so viciously punching the keys because I can not punch—well, where I want to.

A physician, the other day, brought the leader of one of these morbid groups into my room and introduced him to me. The physician's intentions were kindly and considerate. In order to let the visitor know that I had permission to use my typewriter he said. "Mr.—, here, is in an unusual position. He is here practically at his own volition and we are letting him do some writing, as he is a newspaper man."

The visitor took my hand with self-conscious fusiveness. "I am happy to meet you, Mr. ———. You handle a typewriter marvelously. Did you have any experience before you came here? Or have you learned here at the asylum? How interesting. And what were you sent here for? Do you think you are getting better? Do you think you will ever get well enough to get out? Well, so long. See you later."

How unpretty a thing a man is when he lets his curiosity run naked and crass.

We have to have visitors. But they are something like the measles I had as a boy. They make my face hot, they make me break out in a rash, and they make me sick at the stomach. But measles comes only once.

But the visitors are a part of the public. And the public elects legislators and state officers. Legislators make appropriations for state hospitals and some of the state officers are in a position to have much to do with either rutting or greasing the road for hospital authorities if any of "their constituents" are not shown proper courtesies.

Then the visitors may be taxpayers or second cousins of taxpayers. And taxpayers, sir, are titled to free admission to any of the entertainments paid for out of "our money." And chief among the legitimate amusements provided by the state through the medium of "our money" is a trip through the insane asylum, with the creepy thrills incident thereto.

Of course a trip through the penitentiary, or even a reform school, is entertaining too, but the freaks displayed are not of such unusual types.

Not that the physicians like the manners of the crude visitors. I have detected one here looking thoroughly disgusted at some crassness. But they are about as helpless as we are, in such cases. They must be courteous to all visitors, or what a howl there would be! And what charges would flock in to the controlling board or the governor!

And I am again reminded that, unless I have more intestinal stamina than the average man, I should go far, far from my former scenes of activities when I "go home." Otherwise some day when I am heading the community chest campaign to raise funds for the relief of the starving, the sick and the helpless; or while I am publishing editorials intended to teach kindly tolerance for all human frailties and follies, some of these carrion-minded curiosity visitors are quite certain to bob up and say, sneeringly,

"Him? Why I knew him when—"

CHAPTER VII

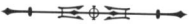

UNRESTRAINED SENSES

THIS has been a red letter day for the patients on the receiving ward. At breakfast this morning every patient had eggs and hot biscuits. On some previous occasions we have had one or the other, but this time we had both. We had plenty of butter and syrup for the hot biscuits, then we had oatmeal and coffee also. What a breakfast!

But the wonder did not cease there. At noon we had ice cream and each man had a tiny square of cake, in addition to the usual black-eyed peas, boiled rice and potatoes. The ice cream was made by patients and had in some way acquired a generous seasoning of salt, but we smacked our lips over it delightedly, and enjoyed it. You see the taste of ice cream is so very unfamiliar here. Nelson, one of our irrepressible wits, held his saucerful up for general inspection and gravely inquired if anyone present could tell him what "this cold stuff" was.

In the outside world eating is either a pleasure, a pastime, or a hurried duty to be attended to in the shortest possible time so that you can get back to work to earn more money so that you can eat again, so that you can earn more money so that Help! Help! I seem to be running around in circles, just like the people outside.

But in an insane asylum eating is one of the chief concerns of every locked-in. The urge to get food is not limited to the insane; it is a cardinal one, primal and ineradicable. It begins with the baby's first cry and ends with the death rattle in the throat. The hurly-burly hodge-podge of civilization has, to some extent, subordinated it to other desires, but it is ineradicably there. Just get yourself marooned on an uninhabited island and see where your first thoughts and efforts will turn. If your curiosity is not that impelling then ask the insane.

In here, inherent instincts are baldly unrestrained. If your reasoning is clouded and you see something on the plate of another man which you want, you are very apt to grab it until taught better by the irate robbed patient or the watchful attendants. Even in this ward where the majority of patients are rational or near-rational a large part of the time, it is a matter of good judgment to reach your place at table before the others have had time to decide whether they want anything you may have on your plate.

For some time after my arrival the physician placed me on a "special diet." In this institution that means that I got one egg each day and soup and milk occasionally. It took me just about two days to discover that if I happened to be the last one to reach my table I was quite apt to find my egg or milk missing and some nearby patient looking self-consciously innocent.

When the door leading to the dining room is opened there is a mad scramble to be the first in line. And—(Shush, please don't mention it)—I have learned to scramble with the rest. But that is just—er—self—self-protection, you understand.

Some of the patients retain a part of the mannerliness which they had outside and so do not grab or filch food from others, but most of them do not hesitate to ask for and pile up on their plates far more food than they can possibly eat. Although the food is drab and monotonous the patients can always get plenty, but that primal food urge is not always restrained by reason, among my present associates.

As for that, I have seen portly captains of industry continue to guzzle steak long after hunger had been succeeded by an overstuffed feeling.

And if you invite a modern lady out for the evening the odds are about three to one that her mental trend will be toward a night club with a surfeit of food and drinks, in spite of the three meals she probably has had during the day.

Hey—quit looking at me with that sarcastic grin—I admit I am in a poor position to be spouting homilies and I tickled my appetite with whiskey until it induced the mad, recurrent craving which brought me here.

The table manners of some of the fellows here are quite entertaining, if you like that sort of entertainment. There is Joe. He has been here twenty years and knows that he has always had sufficient to eat. But at every meal he stealthily will fill his pockets with food—including soupy black-eyed peas.

And Hardeman, who recently was transferred to one of the "untidy" wards, was petulantly particular about how his food should be prepared before he would eat a bite. He would mix together all of the articles of food on his plate, pour his glass of water over them and reduce the whole to a sloppy, swill-like mass. Then he would guzzle it, sonorously, from a tablespoon.

I remember two or three salads, which have been set before me in restaurants, which I have reason to suspect were concocted *à la* Hardeman.

Don't be supercilious. The boys in here are quite like the best people outside except that they are less restrained by conventions and appearances.

It is true that some of them stuff food down their mouths with both hands, steal from the fellow who is not looking, demand or grab more, hoard food in their pockets when they can not eat another bite, and wipe their fingers on their trousers. But don't many of our best people do much the same things in slightly more dainty ways

I do not wipe my fingers on my trousers, but before I start using my knife, fork and spoon I wipe them on the tablecloth. We have no napkins to wipe them with, and I dislike having a black rim around my mouth when I finish eating. The dish-washing is done by patients. The better patients—(Business of prideful preening)—all wipe their knives and forks on the tablecloth.

I should not poke fun at my associates: they have been too kind to me for that. The kindness of many is not to be judged by their manners, mental twists or general dispositions. There is Fred Sells. His mind is so shattered that he can not talk connectedly, his monotonous rattle of conversation hopping from one incoherent subject to another. In the dining room his principal amusement, after his hunger is satisfied, is in throwing bits of food at the other patients until he is sharply stopped. Yet every morning he offers to clean up my room for me; he brings me water when my neuritis keeps me in bed, and several times a day he will come to me to ask solicitously how I am feeling and if there is anything he can do for me.

He has been afflicted with the most pernicious of social diseases for so long that the spirochete, the deadly micro-organism causing that disease, has made its way into his brain. The patients here say that when that happens the mind is always affected and few men ever recover.

This is more or less true. Certain it is that the eradication of the spirochete requires a long and strenuous fight, conducted with the most enlightened medical knowledge. The physicians here do not stop at utilizing mercurial rubs, and intra-muscular and intravenous injections as commonly used outside; they inoculate the patients with the germs of malaria and let the malaria fight the spirochete.

This is a method developed by a German scientist. The patient develops a very high temperature, due to the fever of malaria, and this internal bodily heat attenuates and sometimes kills the spirochete. When the fever is believed to have done its work the malaria is arrested by quinine treatment and the blood and spinal fluid of the patient are tested. If the spirochete infection is overcome the patient improves and sometimes his mental condition becomes such that he is able to go out and resume a place in the workaday world.

Scientists are now working on a plan to produce the same internal bodily heat through electrical devices. This is still in an experimental stage. Perhaps a way may yet be found to fight the pernicious spirochete effectually.

The malarial treatment offers a distinct ray of hope to those afflicted with the forms of insanity which the spirochete causes. Some cures have been reported which are remarkable. But the treatment is still in somewhat of an experimental stage, and in many cases it has failed to restore the patient.

There is an almost universal misconception of how insanity is treated. I know many people, otherwise well informed, who have a hazy impression that physicians have some mysterious knowledge of how to treat the brain to overcome insanity. I believe that no experienced and competent physician ever gives a single dose of medicine in an effort to cure, directly, any form of insanity.

If the mental trouble is the result of any physical malady or condition he tries to remove the physical cause; he then depends upon the recuperative forces of nature to clear up the mind. In this, nature is aided by just four factors: rest, sleep, nutrition and discipline. And the discipline should be even more directed toward permitting and inducing normal thinking than it is toward the control of the patients.

This is why attendants should be conscientious, patient, and mentally capable of thoroughly understanding each individual patient, yet possessed of a firm voice and hand in making patients understand that they must do as they are told to do. Some, a very, very few, are like that.

The wonder is not that most attendants fall far below the qualifications which men in charge of the insane should have; the real wonder is that hospital authorities are able to secure or to train up as high a class of men as they do get. The parsimonious and indifferent attitude of the public toward the insane is to blame for this.

The attendants, when they enter the work, usually get a salary of $35 a month, with room and board thrown in; and $45 a month with room and board is considered a good salary for fully experienced men. Yet they must work an average of 13 hours daily, in constant association with pitifully distorted minds, and take personal physical risks in addition. They must either know or learn something of practical barbering, sanitation, administration of simple medicines, making out numerous reports, and how to seize and hold a struggling patient without hurting him or getting injured.

They should be possessed of a double measure of watchfulness, a triple portion of patience, a working knowledge of psychology sufficient to judge the mental progress of the patient, and enough diplomacy to make him feel that any task assigned him is an indispensable cog in the movement of the world. To round out their qualifications they should be good "kidders." I have seen the charge attendant, here, "kid" patients out of a bad temper, fits of sullenness or irascibility, filthy habits and even little obsessions. He chaffs them until they shamefacedly go off by themselves, ruminate on their own foolishness and adopt a different line of thought. He tells me this method is successful only with those patients who are more or less children in mentality, but that includes many of them.

No wonder some of the attendants themselves sometimes go insane. Oh yes, it has happened. And the attendants sometimes have been confined in the same institutions where they formerly had charge of wards.

Under the present archaic methods of forcibly massing together supersensitive neurasthenics and violent victims of dementia praecox, gentle natured men suffering only from amnesia, and sullen homicidal lunatics—the attendants have far, far more to do with the possible recovery or further deterioration of the minds of the patients than the physicians possibly can have, no matter how capable the doctors may be.

There is usually one physician to each three or four hundred patients. Sometimes the number of patients under one doctor is much larger. Usually the doctor makes two hurried rounds of his wards each day. He has scarcely time to glance at each patient and to exchange a few terse words with those who are called to his attention by the attendants. Frequently he never casts an eye on some of the patients for a week at a time. I believe there are scores of patients whose names and faces the physicians could not associate if suddenly called upon to do so.

Patients often are transferred from one ward to another. If the physician on the new ward did not chance to be present when the patient received his original hearing before the clinic he has no personal knowledge whatever of the patient's peculiarities or needs. Always he must depend upon written and very rudimentary reports from the attendants as to the progress of the patients.

But the patients are under the charge of attendants every hour of the day or night. The charge attendant comes to know his patients as a country teacher knows the pupils in her school room, through continual supervision over them and familiarity with their dispositions.

His opinion, in most cases, can bring a patient before the physicians for inquiry as to his fitness for parole, or have him transferred to a less rational ward. Most important is the fact that all four factors contributing to the recovery of a patient—rest, sleep, nutrition, and discipline—are directly under charge of the attendants.

The effects of the attendants' treatment and handling of the patient are the all important factors in determining whether the mind of the patient will recover—after the physicians have restored his physical health, if this is impaired.

I believe that being confined, year after year, sharpens some senses and creates some habits in a way that nothing else can do. I know the patients develop a marvelous keenness of hearing and practice a cunning system of espionage on everything which happens on the ward.

I sat in my room, one morning, talking with the ward physician. We talked in comparatively low tones. The door into the hall was open but not a patient was in sight. Yet the doctor scarcely had left the ward before one of the patients slipped into my room, retailed almost exactly the conversation I had held with the physician and asked me, suspiciously, what was meant by several statements. He was like many of the others, always reading into everything he saw or heard a double meaning, actuated by sinister motives. Needless to say I have not reported this instance or several more like it which have occurred since. For some reason I have no desire to give this fellow any tenable grounds for believing that I am "spying on him."

Some patient filched a part of this story from my room and I have never recovered it. I suspect Goodner, a tall, middle aged man with a craggy face and smouldering eyes.

He believes that he is relentlessly pursued by "enemies "—wholly imaginary. Several times I have caught him watching me suspiciously as I wrote. One day when both of the attendants were out on the porch he stalked straight to the door of my room.

"Whatchya writing?" he demanded, ominously. My guardian angel was hovering right over me; I happened to be making out the daily ward report. With what was intended to be a sweetly disarming smile, I told him so.

"Lemme see it." He reached right over and pulled it out of my typewriter. His eyes wandered uncomprehendingly over it. He can read but little, but the fact that he had got to see it satisfied him and he surrendered it just as one of the attendants came down the hallway and scurried him back to the day room.

With some of the patients any unusual food dainty is something to hide, to hoard and to protect. They hide fruit or cake which they may receive from home, and eat it by stealth. But many of the others are quite illogically generous. One patient here gave away every piece of candy in a box which he received last Easter. A little later that afternoon I discovered him looking disconsolately out of the window and absent-mindedly testing the strength of the bars.

"Wish I had kep' a piece of that candy," he said regretfully. "Now I can't get any more till my birthday, and I bet I eat every piece of that."

But this generous urge and the ability of the patients to hear when least expected to do so, have their uses; they relieved me of a bad headache, one night. I had developed the headache after the physician had made his afternoon round of the ward so I had no order for medicine. When I asked the attendant for aspirin he refused, as attendants are not permitted to give medicine without orders from the physicians.

I turned out my light and went to bed. A moment later one of the patients slipped silently into my room, handed me two aspirin tablets, placed his finger against his lips to enjoin silence, and slipped out. He had heard the attendant refuse to give me any medicine for my headache, although his room is several doors from mine,

I wondered how he had obtained the aspirin as all medicines are kept carefully locked up. Later I learned how some of the men put over a little scheme on the physician. When one of them has a headache he gets two or three others to help him out, and all of them tell the doctor they have headaches. In this way they sometimes get several tablets and save them secretly for emergencies. They do not consider this a sin—and neither do I. I have several tablets hidden away for the next unexpected headache. Of course patients are not permitted to have medicines in their possession; there are too many dangerous possibilities.

Sunderland, the patient who brought me the aspirin and who has been here for years, proved to me yesterday that there is a bright side to anything if you can only discover it. I was standing at one of the barred windows and made some gloomy remark about always being compelled to look through bars. "I'm glad they have 'em," Sunderland said. "If they didn't have 'em I might go crazy sometime and jump out of the window and kill myself."

He told me that years ago the hospital authorities had tried the plan of leaving the windows on the upper floors unbarred but had been forced to bar them after several patients had jumped out of the high windows, seriously injuring or killing themselves. A physician has since corroborated this.

The patients who jumped illustrated the fact that insane patients often are apt to blunder in trying to escape. They could have tied their bedclothes together and let themselves down to within safe jumping distance of the ground. Evidently they did not think of that. It was too obvious and reasonable.

But since I have learned that the bars are there to protect the insane from themselves as much as to keep us in, they do not depress me so much. If they were not there I might "go crazy" and do a high dive myself; particularly so if I continue to let myself brood about Constance, who refuses to forget me, and to try to puzzle out the conscientious dividing line between the obligation imposed by gratitude and my duty toward myself.

CHAPTER VIII

INSIDIOUS FEARS

THERE was a wild hullabaloo on the ward, the other night, and I got mixed up in it just sufficiently to have that grim old schoolmaster, Experience, add a new chapter to my education.

A new patient had arrived during the afternoon. He must have been a descendant of Goliath, or one of the sons of Anak. He was so huge that he made men of ordinary stature look puny. He stood at least six feet, four inches in height, weighed well over 250 pounds, and had a disconcertingly wide pair of shoulders.

To me he did not appear to be violent, or apt to become violent. His face was lighted up with a religious frenzy and he was shouting, "Praise the Lord, God bless you all, Praise the Lord," with scarcely a pause for breath. His face continually radiated a fanatical light. But he seemed tractable, to my inexperience. I am more experienced now.

The attendants got him to bed with little trouble and got him partially quieted. Bed time came and we all forgot about the huge new patient. I went to sleep fairly early and was paying homage to Morpheus with abandoned devotion. By 11 o'clock snores rose from single rooms and dormitory alike, in a stertorous chorus.

Crash! Smash! From the day hall came alarming sounds which could come from nothing less than a fair sized riot. Shouts, the clatter of falling objects, a wild rushing and the mighty bellows of that religion-crazed giant merged in one mighty uproar.

I dashed madly for the day hall, which is kept lighted all during the night. As I rushed through the doorway from the corridor my eyes, in a flash, took in a tableau which could not be duplicated anywhere in the world except within the walls of an insane asylum.

In the center of the room, his hair disheveled, towered that raving zealot. In one huge hand he brandished a bucket. His other mighty arm was upraised, and with both arm and voice he was abjuring the whole world to give up its sins.

A vase, the flowers which it had contained and the table on which it had stood, had been knocked to the floor. Chairs were overturned and scattered about. The room looked as if a tornado had swept through it.

But it was the human actors in the tableau who caught my eye and made me pause for a moment. That frenzied Goliath had his back to me and was facing one of the parole men who is always the first to rush in and seize a fighting patient. But he was not rushing in this time—not into reach of that brandished bucket in the hands of a frenzy-fired giant. He had snatched up a heavy chair and was holding it up in front of him as a shield to protect his head and body from the threatened blows. The bucket, swung by that arm, could have crushed a skull.

Back of the huge man three other "trusty" patients were grouped, but they were standing as though glued to their tracks. In the hasty glance which I swept over them I saw that not one of them wanted to be the first to dash into grips with the man. They were not exactly terrified—but no one was making a move. I noticed that the jaw of one of them had dropped until his mouth hung open. The other two were plainly trying to think out some safe plan of attack.

In the second that I stood there, taking in the scene, an old trick, learned on the football field years ago, flashed into my mind. If I had taken a second thought I feel sure that I would not have had the grit to try it, but I did not wait to think. I launched myself in a flying tackle, like a catapult bolt, straight at the small of that mighty back, one shoulder hunched forward for the shock, my legs flexed for the next move.

As my shoulder struck his back with all of my weight and the power of my dive behind it I wrapped both of my legs about the ankles of the big man. No one less than a superman can stand upright against an unexpected charge of this kind. My drive threw the patient off his balance, and my legs, twined and locked about his ankles, prevented his throwing either foot forward to regain it. He crashed forward toward the floor. Goliath had gone down under a surprise attack.

Then I had plenty of help. The four men who had stood frozen a moment before, had hold of him before he fairly hit the floor. Others dashed in from both doors. And they all were needed. Still praising the Lord, as he flailed out with his great arms and legs in a paroxysm of fanatical zeal and fighting frenzy, that religious maniac put up a struggle on the floor that will be long remembered here.

He was buried under overwhelming numbers. The night attendant dashed in from the hallway. Another attendant rushed up from the ward beneath ours. The bucket was torn from the patient's grasp, but it took two men to handle that one arm and accomplish the trick. A strait-jacket was forced on him. He was lifted into bed by a dozen men, tied down and rendered helpless. Then attendants and patients backed away to take account of bruises and scratches.

The zealot, while that struggle went on, never ceased his exhortations. "Praise the Lord; Give up your sins and come unto Me," roared his booming voice. "This is God's night; Praise the Lord," he was shouting "God will bless you all," while he was doing his level best to bash heads. When, jacketed and pinioned, he was lifted into bed he looked about the room, now crowded with frightened patients, and his face lighted up with pleasure. "It's a great night for the Lord," he said. "You are all here. It's a house full for the Lord; How He will rejoice; It's a full house for the Lord. Praise the Lord."

As for me, the moment that Son of Anak tumbled and the others piled in I rolled clear and sat up. I wanted to count my own bruises. I had thrown my arms around him as my hurtling shoulder struck the small of his back, and when his huge bulk crashed against the floor I had skinned an elbow, beautifully. Then, even while he was falling, he had snatched one of his legs free and, with toes spread wide, he had "clawed" me with the toenails of that foot. The legs of my pajamas had prevented the toenails going in deep, but my shin had been scratched from the knee nearly to the ankle.

After it was all over I learned why the other patients had hesitated to attack the man. It was not altogether his size and the brandished bucket. They would have dashed in on almost any other type of patient but experience has taught them that of all the classes of insane the most dangerous are the religious maniacs.

"You never know when one of these fellows will believe that the Lord has told him to kill all the sinful people in the world, and he always tries to carry out God's commands," one of the attendants told me. Other insane patients have an actual dread of the religious fanatics. Such patients are not governed by the considerations which keep other classes of patients within the control of the attendants. They have no physical fear whatever while their religious frenzy is on them. They seem exalted by the belief that they are doing God's will and, for the time being, fear simply is not in them. They believe they are headed straight for Heaven, in any event, so why should they be afraid to die?

They took the giant to the Hydro. This department of the hospital is arranged and equipped to administer hydrotherapeutic treatments. "Packing" is the treatment most used. The patients are wrapped in sheets, from neck to feet. Then the sheets are drenched with water and blankets are wrapped around the swathed patients.

The treatment causes a condition of heavy perspiration, and the long periods in the packs have a physically weakening and mentally quieting effect which often brings violent patients out of their paroxysms.

Patients who are in a violent or badly disturbed condition when first brought in often are sent to the Hydro after being checked in and remaining on the receiving ward for a day or two of observation. Some of them afterward become very tractable patients. The mental fever which causes the paroxysm seems to be relieved. My friend Goliath, after a week in the Hydro, seems to be making a slight improvement. At least he is not preaching so often or so vociferously.

Inmates who have never been confined in the Hydro have a wholesome fear of being transferred to it. They do not understand it, so they fear it. They believe that patients sent there are packed in ice and allowed to nearly freeze. They believe the unfortunates can not sleep for weeks at a time, and they say that when patients get to screaming, pitchers of ice water are dashed into their faces until they are nearly strangled to death.

This latter statement has some basis in fact. Attendants and physicians have learned that a pitcher of cold water dashed into the face of a screaming patient often will quiet him, without injuring him, when nothing else will do so. I know this plan is used at times.

I believe that attendants do not want to correct the false impression that patients have about the Hydro. It is good judgment to have one "bogey man" to hold before the patients as a deterrent against unruliness. I have heard them warn men that if they did not stop being troublesome they would be sent to the Hydro, and I never heard one of them tell a patient just how the dreaded Hydro is conducted. Those who have been confined there for a time have learned about it and do not fear it.

In the minds of every one of the insane persons with whom I have come in contact there is one emotion which overshadows and outweighs all other activities of their minds. It is fear; fear which no effort of their will can overcome or dislodge; unreasoning fear, often vague and formless but hopelessly controlling and impelling.

Most physicians probably will disagree with me in this, but I believe the faint and almost indistinguishable line of demarcation between sanity and insanity is the point where fear gets beyond the possibility of control by any effort of the will or other mental faculties.

The man who is recognized as sane controls his fears to such an extent that he does not permit them to overwhelm or sweep away his reasoning. Whenever he lets his fears sweep away his reasoning he is qualified to join those of us who are already here.

I believe the familiar saying, "gone mad with fear," is unintentionally a statement of scientific fact.

Many patients try to hide their obsessionary fears from the physicians and attendants, fearing that if they are found out they will never be permitted to go home. Those most nearly sane try to conceal them from the other patients also, but their conversation in unguarded moments almost invariably betrays them. To the insane their obsessionary fears are not fears; they are stark, incontrovertible realities, so indisputably real that any arguments which other persons may offer against them are simply silly, and the person who advances them is a hopeless fool—or insane.

Fears of the insane are almost never physical. Usually insane people have little physical fear; sometimes none at all which can be detected. Their fears are those which lurk in the mind; obsessions are largely fears or the result of fears.

Even in the religious maniacs their fear that they may not be "saved," or may displease or fail to please the Jehovah is the actuating motive for their actions, I believe.

Suicidals fear life itself or some of its problems. Melancholiacs fear their own thoughts, introspections or self-judgments. Some of the insane fear that they are pursued by enemies. My belief is that homicidals are actuated by fear; not by a wanton desire to slay. They fear some mysterious something or some one and they kill to remove the source of that fear.

Some of the fears of the insane are not obsessionary, though they may arise from the patient's obsessions or other mental conditions. Epileptics fear that they will have convulsions. Many patients live in continual fear of the return of their disturbed periods. Some fear, oh how they fear, that they will never recover.

Some patients fear to go back into the outside world. There are two patients on this ward who are apparently entirely recovered. The physicians are willing to release them, but they are afraid to leave. One says he can not force himself to face people who know that he has been insane; the other says he fears a recurrence of his former insanity. I believe he is really afraid that he can not make good outside.

A very few of the patients are afraid of death but this fear is secondary; what they really fear is that death may come before they can get discharged from the hospital. They want to "go home."

Even the man here who is "always right" and who is violently angry with any one who fails to agree with him, really is actuated by fear. Let the bigots outside deny that and I will offer proofs. But they won't do it because real bigots won't admit their bigotry. They are always right.

I won't attempt to analyze my own fears. I am not sure what my dominant fear is. It may be that I am afraid to decide between my obligations to Constance and my ambitions for myself.

Perhaps I am limiting the matter too much in believing that the uncontrollability of fear marks the thin and indistinguishable line between sanity and insanity. At least one of the physicians here believes that I am. He holds that when any of the emotions become so turgid or great that they pass beyond the control of judgment or reason, the dividing line between sanity and insanity is passed.

How I would be comforted if I could just agree with him fully. That definition reaches out and includes most of the inhabitants of this big, round world. I am not personally acquainted with any of the inhabitants of Mars or the other planets, but I strongly suspect that it includes them, also.

That definition would make the only difference between those of us who are locked in and those who are permitted to carry on untrammeled in the great outside, the difference lying in the fact that those of us who are here have been detected in our aberrations while those outside have so far escaped. I feel much better already, thank you.

Under that definition I have seen 50,000 insane persons at one running of the Kentucky derby. As the straining thoroughbreds came thundering down the home stretch I believe there were fully half a hundred thousand men and women who could not have told you at the moment what state they hailed from, or even what their names were. What do little things like that matter in those reason-snatching last ten seconds, when you are screaming, begging, praying for some particular one of these gallant horses to "Come on, Boy. Come on." Reason has been kicked flying out of the grandstand; emotion has full control and is running stride for stride with the horses, just then. If you have been there you will remember that reason came back slowly and hesitatingly, as though it was not quite sure of its welcome. In all honesty, were you quite sure that you wanted to descend from the maddening thrill of the moment?

Fine. Come right on in and join us. You will feel perfectly at home. So there.

And what about the spectators at a prize fight or a wrestling match, when rabid fans are howling, "Kill him. Knock his block off. Pull an arm off of him," and such usual pleasantries? Are those fans able to say they are not suffering a temporary attack of insanity?

I remember seeing a lady—pardon me, a woman—dash her cards into the face of her partner when he made a stupid play at bridge. He was not her own husband, so she did not feel at liberty to shoot him. And I have seen the New York Stock Exchange suffering from the stark frenzy of a hundred thousand speculators, and I feel sure that their emotions had got completely out of the control of their reasoning. Let's diagnose their mental trouble as emotional insanity, and confine all speculators for fear they may have another "disturbed spell" and bring financial misery on millions of innocent bystanders. That is what they have done to those of us who are already here; they have locked us up for fear that when we are "not normal" we may do an injury to some one else. Yet I can not imagine how it would be possible to cause more widespread injury to others during a "disturbed spell" than just to permit the speculators to bring about another stock market crash. I believe I am beginning to like the doctor's definition.

But how about the fellows who would scorn the thought that they were insane yet who would flatly refuse to walk under a ladder or to continue on down a smooth highway if a black cat should chance to cross in front of them? They can not have the comfort of claiming that their delusions and obsessions are temporary; those delusions usually stick fast for a lifetime. Their deluded spells never give them a respite.

I know a very successful business man on the outside who would gasp and turn pale with horror if he should happen to break a mirror, and he would be hesitating and afraid to make any important move until some sort of "bad luck" happened. Then he would feel that the god of mischance had been appeased for the heinous crime of breaking the mirror, and he could lift up his head and smile in confidence once more.

Does the fact that he is successful in business absolve him from the charge that he has delusions? Well, as for that, the man who has the room directly across the hallway from my own room, in this hospital for the insane, is the owner of one of the most pretentious department stores in a large city.

The executor of his estate says he is worth a million dollars. He retains all of his business acumen. For years he was considered merely eccentric, but sane because he was successful in business. Then he became too successful. His wealth attracted avaricious eyes, His "eccentricities" were scrutinized, and he was declared insane. He has been locked up here for ten years, but through his friendly executor he has kept a hand on his business and it is still growing. He is insane, but I know a good many allegedly level headed men who would wager that he could go out today, start from scratch, and beat the average business man in getting together a new fortune. Just who are the insane, anyway, under the doctor's definition?

Faugh. It has been a wearying day, and that has made me cynical and snarly. Spring has given way to summer; hot, wilting, deadening summer; doubly deadening to those of us who are shut up within four walls. All day the men have been irritable and sullen. Even the flies and cockroaches have seemed to be more plentiful and pestiferous. There is not a fly-swatter on the ward, so we slap at the flies with our hands. We wage unceasing war on the cockroaches, but they are like the poor, they are always with us.

They seem to have a fellow feeling for those other bugs, the insane. Men who have been confined in other institutions tell me that they are always riotously prevalent in insane asylums.

For several hours I have fumed and stewed, crabbedly trying to pound my typewriter to help kill the stifling time. Women in the ward across the court have been screaming all day. They will shriek all night. It must be hell in the violent wards today. And tonight will be hell for all the patients in all of those wards where the inmates are locked in their rooms through all the long, hot nights from dusk until the rising hour. We who are more fortunate can keep the doors and windows of our rooms and the windows of the halls open, and thus can get a little draft. Of course when we have the windows open there are still the double bars. But, thank goodness, whatever little breeze there is can find its way between the bars—and how it helps.

But those who are locked in their tiny, close rooms have but one window, and it usually opens on a court. Their clothes are taken away from them when they are locked in, to prevent their attempting to escape during the night, but in weather such as this they should not mind that.

I wonder if it is "stir fever" which is binding me to such a nasty mood? Or is it that I have been mulling over a problem that I have to face in regard to Constance, the woman back home who declines to forget me.

Oh well, there is a dance tonight; the last one till cooler weather comes in the fall. I think I will go, and watch the dancing of the girl in the red party dress. Perhaps it will give me something to think about which will jerk me out of my depressive self-analysis.

I hope it will drive the constancy of Constance out of my mind.

CHAPTER IX

Pot Pourri

I HAVE learned about the girl in the red party dress, only she did not wear it at the dance last night. She wore one of the dresses made in the hospital sewing room. She may have made it herself from materials supplied by the state. I suspect her red dress is about worn out, and I also suspect that she regrets its passing. She had a downcast air. But that did not detract from the gracefulness of her dancing.

Her story? The grim pity of it! That young girl—she is only twenty-two—came here a confirmed alcoholic, like myself. She has been here three years. She learned to drink at high school parties. She wanted to be up-to-the minute, like the other girls, and her boy friends. But she is of the nervous, sensitively high-strung type; the type which people who are not too well informed or too nicely discriminating refer to as neurotic. She is just the sort of person in whom alcohol sets the fangs of periodic mental craving in a very brief time.

With men and women of this type so brief is the time and so insidious is the clamping down of the mental habit that the victims scarcely ever realize the danger until the periodically recurring craving is deeply enchanneled in the brain. Only time can cure that—time in which nature may erase a brain scar.

The mental craving is wholly different and separable from the physical desire for alcohol. The various "liquor cures" can eradicate the physical desire for alcohol within a few days; but they can not possibly reach into the brain and extract a periodic mental craving any more than physicians can cure other forms of insanity by medicines administered internally.

Don't I know? Haven't I spent thousands of dollars on liquor cures and psychopathic hospitals in a dozen states? But that is a different story. What I learned about this girl jerked that digression out of my mind and tumbled it down upon my typewriter keys.

Joan, yes that is her name, was driven by restless nervous energy in everything she ever did. No matter what she undertook she had to excel others. In her studies she led her classes. She was the life of the party at every gathering of her boy and girl friends. If the skirts of the other girls were short, hers must be shorter. If the other girls "necked" she must neck more abandonedly. If the other girls took a drink—and they did—she must take two drinks—and she did.

Her father voted for prohibition, and kept plenty of liquor in his automobile-sales office to put prospective customers in a good humor. Her mother kept a supply at home to liven up bridge parties because it was being done; everybody was doing it, in fact everybody expected it.

Joan played bridge. She played well because she must excel in every thing. She excelled also in drinking liquor.

In public utterances her father approved the Volstead law. It kept working men from soaking themselves with liquor and abusing or starving their families. Sure it was a good thing. It made the cost of liquor pretty high and the quality bad, but it was a good thing for the working man.

Yes, in public, he approved the law; the law that put shrewd young bootleggers, backed by older men, into high school classes and college fraternity houses; that law that made the boy who went to parties a back number if he did not have a flask on his hip; that law that made a sixteen-year-old girl a wallflower if she could not toss off her whiskey neat.

The inevitable happened. Joan, with a great deal of secrecy, was bundled off to a liquor cure in a distant city. The neighbors must not know, even as they drank their liquor over the bridge tables in her parents' home. She stayed a month, and was sent home free of the physical craving but with that mental craving, driven by jangled nerves, setting her wild.

That periodic craving had crashed through her weakened defenses.

But the family must not be disgraced. Her parents must not suffer the humiliation of having a liquor addict for a daughter. They conspired with the family physician. He drew a neat sum in fees from them during the course of a year, so could be trusted to help. Joan was committed here— under utmost secrecy of course. It must not be known. It might disrupt the bridge club or hurt the sale of an automobile.

"Yeah, she came here three years ago," said the parole man who told me about her, at the dance. It extends beyond the uncanny how some of the patients learn all about the others, and remember it in detail. I have been bowled off my pins at discovering how much some of them know about me. But they do not mind baldly asking any other patient all about himself and it is impossible to rebuff them.

"She went home once," the parole man amplified. "But in about three months her folks brought her back; fuller'n a tick, and seein' snakes. They don't want her at home any more and won't help her get out. She isn't crazy. She is just as sane as I am."

I did not smile at that last statement. This patient is one of those who believe they are fully sane. Most of them are not. He isn't.

But I had better be careful in saying such things. Some of the people outside might draw the wrong conclusion about me. They believe that all insane believe all other people insane. Even some doctors have told me that. My experience is that at least half of them are startlingly good judges of the sanity or degree of insanity of their associates or of any one else except themselves. Only certain types believe all others insane.

I presume Joan's mother is still serving cocktails and complaining at the high cost of bootleg liquor. Her father probably is offering each visitor to his office a drink of "pretty good stuff" and not troubling to note who is around.

When his stenographer brings his letters he probably offers her a drink. It is being done; or it was before I was locked in.

As for Joan, she can't carry her liquor, so she will have to remain locked in, legally insane, unless her parents relent, or some friend comes to her assistance; and they have all probably forgotten her. No wonder her eyes are sombre even when she dances.

She can dance round dances only, with a girl for a partner, as long as she remains here. She can have only women associates. She is twenty-two. By the time she is seventy-five she will have been here fifty-six years. She really ought to be used to this sort of life by that time. That's that.

There are not a great many alcoholics among the 2,000 patients here. The institution does not admit them if the authorities discover in advance that they are suffering only from physical alcoholism. Otherwise the hospital would be swamped with them, under prohibition. Periodic alcoholics, those who have developed the recurrent craving, are classed as dipsomaniacs and are admitted. I am told there are more of these coming in than there were in the days of the open saloon.

A few drug addicts are admitted here but most of them are sent to other hospitals. Drug and liquor addicts are given "the iron treatment" here. That means they are not given decreasing amounts of their stimulant on which to "taper off" but are entirely deprived of it from the time they are checked in unless their heart action becomes so weak that a small amount of the drug or alcohol is required to keep them alive. Poor devils!

I am not going to discuss that. I ——

I had been in a private psychopathic hospital for weeks before being sent here. Thank my guardian angels for that.

Here the new patients are nearly all insane from other causes than drugs or liquor. Of these there is a constant stream. Some are far gone in physical weakness when they arrive.

These are the ones who go most often to the paupers' cemetery of the hospital. Some die the day they are received. Perhaps if they had been committed sooner their lives could have been saved. The fever of mental fires has burned up their physical reserves before they are brought to the hospital, trussed up, by peace officers who know little, and perhaps care less, for the difference between dangerous criminals and the tormented insane.

"We can't save them if they are as good as dead when we receive them," one of the attendants told me. He is right. Seared by the crossfire of a tortured mind and a sapped physical vitality, many of these patients die before the recuperative measures of the physicians and attendants can have feet.

That is not the fault of the hospital authorities. But people who do not know the facts are apt to remember only that the patient died after he was brought here. Many such patients have been confined in unsanitary jails for days or weeks, waiting for dilatory officials to find it convenient to get around to their cases. Frequently, very frequently, they come in swarming with vermin to add to their other troubles.

But many times men apparently in the most robust physical condition are killed by their hallucinations. If that be medical heresy, let the reactionary members of the medical profession be stationed for a time in an insane asylum.

There was Goliath, the huge religious zealot who wrecked the day hall, one night. The Gray Wagon came for him. When he came in he seemed to be in the pink of physical condition. He was but forty-three years old. He was sent to the Hydro. He was given good care and at first it was believed that he would recover.

But his rending religious frenzy burnt up the vitality of even that great frame.

And the Concrete Man is gone also. The Gray Wagon made another trip. Death ended his delusion that he was doomed to live for a thousand years. I wonder if he is glad at the release. He had sought death by physical means; he achieved it through a state of mind. His hallucination that he was solid concrete from the neck down prevented his body assimilating the food which the attendants forcibly fed him. His mind finally starved him to death.

Yes indeed; the mind which motivates and regulates bodily functions can as readily wreck them. Those of us who live among the insane see that demonstrated almost daily; demonstrated beyond cavil or question. Wreck that part of your brain which motivates the heartbeat and the heartbeat stops, whether the weapon is a bullet or an hallucination.

While those on the outside are arguing as to whether the mind can cause or cure organic troubles, we on the inside are unalterably convinced that it can. We do not know whether a conscious effort of the will can do so, but most of us believe that it can, at least to some extent.

Even scoffers on the outside might became convinced that the mind does control bodily health if they analyzed their own experiences. A violent and uncontrolled anger often causes biliousness. The fear caused by suddenly looking down from a great height makes many people vomit. The sight of a human body infested with lice will start most people to scratching. A photograph of golden rod will bring on an attack of hay fever in some victims of that peculiar malady. Can not hallucinations hampering some brain center kill a patient as effectively as some drug which acts on the same part of the brain?

We believe so when we see strong men die in violent paroxysms while calmer minded insane continue to live on.

But John Doe lived. Nobody knows John Doe's real name. He was picked up in my home city; his mind was an absolute blank, his body wasted terribly from lack of food. No one could identify him. The newspaper reporters jumped on the story with a vim. In doing so they nearly sealed his fate.

They headlined him as "The Mystery Man." Morbid and interested people by the hundreds flocked in to see him or to try to identify him. This kept him in jail for several days, and county jailers know little about feeding and caring for such mindless persons. When he was brought to the hospital his spark of life was near the flickering point. And vermin crawled over him.

Physicians and attendants probably swore at the task in front of them but they went to it with a vim. They put up a determined fight for that wavering existence. Twice daily his clenched teeth were pried apart with a wooden wedge, and milk and raw eggs, beaten together, were fed him through a rubber tube, extending into his stomach. The wedge had to be kept between his teeth during the feeding to prevent his teeth closing on the tube and severing it. The vermin were routed. Stimulants were administered. Slowly his body began to mend. He never spoke. He made no conscious movements, even with his eyes. They were vacant, almost lifeless.

When his strength grew to the point where he might safely be moved he was transferred to one of the hospital wards. He is still John Doe; with a buried past, and relatives unknown.

But as one outstandingly queer patient leaves the receiving ward, either feet first or between two attendants, another takes his place. There's the Spider, who has been here but a few days.

The Spider gets his nickname from trying to climb the walls. If he can avoid the eyes of watchful attendants and trusty patients he will climb up on the gratings which cover the insides of the windows.

Clinging with fingers and toes, hands and feet wide spread, for all the world like a big spider, he will run across or up the window grating till some one pulls him down. He will try to climb the blank walls. He does not seem to know why he feels impelled to climb, but climb he does at every opportunity. He is apparently harmless—but the other patients and the attendants say shortly, "look out for that type of man."

Then there is Jazzy. I don't know his other name. Few of the patients do. He never says anything to anyone. His face shows that he has been an intelligent and educated man. Now it is as vacant as a ghost-guarded house in a southern Negro community, than which nothing could be more vacant. He can not find his way down to the dining room for his meals. Some of the other patients lead him down, seat him at the table and later lead him back to the ward. Apparently he knows almost nothing. He has no memory, even for orders of the attendants. A dozen times a day some one will have to lead him out of the hallway back to his chair in the big day room.

But when anyone wants music he leads Jazzy to the piano and seats him at the stool. Hesitatingly Jazzy's hands find their way to the keys. Sometimes the other patients must put his hands to the keys. But at the first sound of the instrument something in the hidden recesses of his brain seems to respond. There is no light in his eyes, no flicker of memory in his countenance; he does not even look at the instrument.

But as if impelled by some force of which he is not conscious his fingers travel lightly over the keys. Old familiar airs, jazzy dance music, religious tunes, jigs and snatches of classical compositions flow from the keyboard, in no order or sequence and with apparently no volition on his part. Reason, judgment, memory, comprehension—all seem to have fled into some dark limbo, but the tinkle of the piano sets off a spark in some remaining motivating fragment of the mind he once had.

He will continue to play, entirely at random, until some one leads him away from the piano and places him in a seat. At night when he is led to his bed he displays another inexplicable trait. He can undress himself and get into bed unaided. And he can bathe himself when led to the bath tub. These are the only things which he seems to comprehend.

But they are not all vacant minded and harmless, these new patients. Some of them have all the "harmlessness" of a raging wildcat, when aroused. And some of them are possessed of a tricky cunning which is far more deadly than the frenzy of the raging ones.

It was one of the trickily cunning ones who came near being beaten to death by outraged fellow patients on the ward just below this, a few days ago. No incident that ever occurred in an insane asylum could better prove the truth of three truisms which attendants and older patients know by heart. They might almost be called the three "R's" of controlling the insane. They are:

When a patient is unusually quiet for a period, watch him. Don't let him get a chance at you.

No attendant can maintain discipline or even be safe without the good will and aid of the better patients on his ward.

Never go into a patient's room without having him where you can watch him.

One of the attendants on the ward below this is a pleasant faced and good natured young man. He is one of those classed as "good attendants" by the patients. They are not all so classed. Certainly not.

The other morning a patient named Martin, who had been unusually quiet for several days, came to this attendant and told him that his bed was over-run with bedbugs. The attendant should have been wary because while flies and cockroaches are numerous and gregarious here, bedbugs are scarcely known. Then, too, Martin had been unusually quiet.

But the attendant is of anything but a suspicious nature. He is friendly and goes out of his way to do little kindnesses. This trait both jeopardized and saved his life.

He went into Martin's room, letting Martin follow him in. As he stooped over and started to examine the mattress Martin suddenly whipped an improvised slug from his pocket and struck the attendant a crashing blow on the side of the head, knocking him to the floor.

The blow landed with a sharp crack. This and the noise of the attendant's fall to the floor told the patients in the hall that something was wrong. They dashed for the room. Martin, in the meantime, had aimed two more blows at the attendant's head, but while the attendant was badly dazed he was not quite unconscious and he managed to protect his head with his arms. Then the charging patients reached the scene.

Martin was snatched from over his victim, hurled to the floor and the enraged patients swarmed over him. No weapons were needed or wanted. In dealing out retribution in a case of this kind nothing will satisfy the avengers except natural weapons; their hands and their feet. The other attendant dashed out of the day hall and threw himself into the struggling mass of men. An attendant from our ward heard the fierce commotion and dashed down. Together the attendants, largely through the weight of authority, rescued Martin and quieted the vengeful patients. They were just in time. The other patients had nearly done for him.

"If we'd a had about two minutes more he'd been the deadest man you ever saw," one of the patients told me later. "I'd helped kill him myself, if I could a got hold of him, but there was too many on him."

And that last statement explains just why Martin was not dead when the attendants jerked him out from under choking hands and trampling feet. The avenging patients got in each other's way. As it was he had to be taken to a hospital ward, badly beaten.

The attendant was treated for head cuts and contusions and was back on duty by the afternoon of the same day. Some of these young fellows have a generous admixture of what the army boys call "guts," even if they did get most of their growth during the post-war jazz age. Make no mistake about that.

One of the physicians, later, explained to me how the attendant managed to retain consciousness after the first blow. "The realization that he faced certain death if he yielded to unconsciousness came to him in a flash and kept some part of his brain active," the doctor said. "He fought off unconsciousness until the other patients got there, then he yielded." That seems logical; the attendant was fully unconscious when lifted from the floor.

The slug which the patient used showed how long and cunningly he had planned his attack on the attendant. In the toe of a sock he had placed two iron nuts from the steam radiator pipes, and a polished hardwood block, one of those used in place of casters in the bottom of bedposts, here. Then he tied a knot in the sock, holding the nuts and block tightly in the toe. Swung by a frenzied arm this made a formidable weapon.

He had no tools to remove the nuts from the pipes. They are all so tightly set that it had been believed impossible to remove them with anything less than a long handled wrench. Yet he got them off with his hands. Just how long he was in accomplishing this nobody knows, but it must have taken him several days.

He has admitted that his plan was to knock out the attendant, seize the keys and escape. He would very probably have succeeded had not the fact that this attendant was popular with the patients upset his plans. They would not tolerate a cowardly attack on a man they liked.

Of course this did not include all the patients. It was noticeable that several of the more unruly ones did not join in the rescue of the attendant. These were probably hoping that Martin would succeed in getting the door unlocked and give them an opportunity to get out and make a run for freedom. Yet not one of them was in a mental condition to escape quick detection on the outside. And they had no place to go to find a hiding place, no employment, or friends to assist them. This is true of so very many of the patients. Even their relatives are afraid of them. Criminals very often have friends ready to give them every assistance, even at risks to themselves. Inmates of a hospital who escape are marked and hunted men, though they may be sane. They have been adjudged insane and everyone is afraid they may be.

Here in the hospital we know that it is the new patient just received or one who has been here a long time and has developed "stir fever" who is most apt to display violence towards the attendants. We never know when some of the patients may become angered and violent toward the other patients.

Relatives and the officers who bring them are directly responsible for the fact that many patients are ready to fight when first received. In order to get them here quietly relatives or officers frequently resort to telling them that they are being taken to a hotel or to a general hospital. When they find they are in an insane asylum and locked in they make frantic efforts to escape. Usually they try violence first.

The minute the door is locked behind them they usually realize they have been tricked. Then things begin to happen. Or the first order given them by an attendant may set them off. They have not been accustomed to obeying orders; their relatives or those associated with them have been afraid to give them orders and have depended on wheedling or cajoling them.

Attendants don't wheedle. The first thing a patient must learn is that he is under discipline. The first order he gets is to take a bath. Some of them raise their hackles and refuse. Some of them do not wait to do that; they just start fighting. And that is poor policy; also bad judgment.

A big strapping, husky patient was brought in recently. He came from the mountain section of the state. He and his brothers had been engaged in moonshining in the hill fastnesses. But he had fallen victim of his own wares, complicated by a sullen disposition. He had become deranged, and was brought here. And he was just the type of mountaineer who has never acknowledged any discipline.

He realized where he was being brought and I believe he had made up his mind to start trouble at the first opportunity. He argued insultingly with the attendant who brought him from the main office to the receiving ward, but did not get fully into a fighting mood until he was led into the receiving ward and the door locked behind him. The attendant ordered him to take a bath and that strapping mountaineer started for the attendant. He could have made no worse choice of an attendant to start in on.

It happens that this attendant, who is one of the regular ones on this ward, has been selected by the physicians for the delicate task of bringing in new patients because he has two outstanding qualifications: an even tempered, quiet judgment, and a trained and powerful physique.

When the patient started at him he dodged, "necked" the big fellow and went to the floor with him. Quite often this will take all the fight out of new patients. This time it did not. That mountaineer's mother never raised any children who submitted tamely to anything.

That strapping fellow fought with frenzy, too great a frenzy to enable him to do any clear thinking. Besides he was badly outnumbered.

Another attendant and half a dozen patients piled into the fray. He found his arms twisted behind his back and pinioned, his legs drawn up behind him, and his body pinned to the floor by the neck hold of the attendant, supplemented by the two hundred pound weight of a big patient who was calmly sitting on his abdomen.

He had not been more than scratched, but he was helpless, in spite of frantic struggles until his strength gave out. He had managed to tear a shirt or two off the wearers but had done no real damage. He had simply encountered a sort of force to which he was not accustomed.

Then, while he was held there, the charge attendant told him that there was just one thing he could do, and that was to make up his mind to submit gracefully to hospital discipline. He thought that over, sullenly, for several minutes, then promised to do as he was ordered. The men let him up and he went quietly and took a bath. He has given no trouble since, but the attendants say that he will do so when he becomes restless at confinement, so they are having him transferred to a ward where discipline is more strict than on the receiving

"I know that type of man," the charge attendant told me. "He is not through, yet; not by a long shot. But the next time he will scheme and wait until he can get the advantage."

The attendant who met his rush never said a word while the struggle was under way—and never loosened his hold. He left the giving of orders to the charge attendant. His business was to see that the patient did not hurt either himself or anyone else. He attended to that.

He is much respected and liked by the patients on the ward. He has the reputation of being pleasant and just. "But you don't want to try to put anything over on him," the patients tell the newcomers.

His father died when he was just a boy and he found himself the principal support of his mother, brother and sisters.

He took any work he could get, including working as a section hand almost before he was ready for long pants. He saw his brother and sisters grow up, then he started to educate himself. He has done it well. He married a school teacher, took a teachers' examination, passed with credit, and will teach school this winter. I admire that fellow.

But I hate to see him leave this ward. We do not know just what sort of fellow we may get in his place. We might be unfortunate and get a "hospital bum."

Every hospital gets them. Most of them do not last long. But while they are on the job they can make the usual insane-hospital life far, far worse for the patients. Every patient who has been here very long knows gentry of this class, and dreads them.

Hospital bums, as the patients designate them, are drifting, irresponsible attendants who move from hospital to hospital, always looking for a "softer spot" or just drifting because they are drifters. One who was formerly here had worked in six hospitals in one year. Such fellows usually last just long enough at a hospital to get sufficient cash to take them to the next one.

They know enough about insane-hospital work to deceive the superintendents and supervisor for awhile, but they don't deceive the patients for a minute. The patients usually have such a man tagged as a "bum" by the end of his first day on the ward. They are very seldom wrong.

The only ambition of the hospital bum seems to be to have three meals a day, a place to sleep and cigarette money. He does not study his patients, because he cares nothing about their welfare. Compassion, fairness or kindness are not parts of his mental make up.

It is fellows of this ilk who are responsible for the stories of brutality on the part of attendants which sometimes find their way into the papers.

A flagrant case of unmitigated brutality generally becomes known and the newspapers seize on it avidly. Since such stories are about the only ones concerning hospital life which find their way into the papers the average reader is apt to believe that patients are knocked down, shackled in solitary, trampled or strung up by the thumbs as a matter of daily schedule.

The real tragedies of life in an insane hospital are completely overlooked. The pitifully slow march of long years, devoid of any real hope, the forced association with distorted minds only, the complete absence of understanding companionship of any kind, lifelong lack of association with the other sex, the massing together of all types of the mentally afflicted, the fear of never regaining a free place among fellowmen or respected standing in the eyes of anyone—these never find a place in the general conception of the horrors of life in an insane asylum.

As for me, I almost have reached the point where I would welcome a lively beating as a temporary break in the monotony. At least I would have the pleasure of being very angry about it, brooding over it and hating the man responsible, and otherwise escaping for a time from my doldrums and my ceaseless mulling over the question of what is my conscientious duty, and wisest policy, toward Constance when I go home, and my growing uncertainty as to whether I will have the grit to go back and face my world, the world which knows me, and lick it into re-accepting me.

Fiddlesticks! I wonder what sort of complex I am acquiring. I find myself being snappish with the other patients quite often. I associate with them less and less, sticking close in my little room about twenty-two hours out of the twenty-four; avoiding them, dreading to have them come in and disturb me, hesitating to force myself to overlook their quirks and vagaries and forgive their crudities, for which they are not to blame.

Psychoanalysts call that state of mind a dread complex or dread neurosis, and hint, encouragingly, that the fellow who gives way to it is teeter-tottering at the top of a steep hill down which a greased slide leads straight to paranoia. I had better hop right off my teeter-totter and trot out and mingle with the other patients, listen to and approve their obsessions, rejoice with them in their never ending belief that they will soon be released and go home, and shake off my growing antipathy—not as a matter of kindness but in cold blooded mental self-defense. I don't want to slide down hill into paranoia.

I remember reading a heavily didactic work by some psychoanalyst who said that genuine hearty laughter is the very best cure for such a state of mind. Then my cure is right to my hand. I have only to mingle with the new patients as they come in. Practically every one of them gives me a hearty chuckle—and the most sincere compliment that I ever received.

Until they learn that I am merely "one of the bugs" nearly every one of them will address me as "Doctor." You see they realize that I am not one of the attendants; I am middle aged and not athletic enough for an attendant, and in addition I do not wear a white coat. And, Ahem, excuse my blushing. They think I look too intelligent to be a patient, so they naturally call me Doctor.

I have not told the "other" doctors this yet. I have not studied out their complexes. I might get another chuckle. And I might get a mentally appraising look.

Oh, well. ____?

CHAPTER X

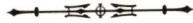

SLEEPING SICKNESS

THE charge attendant has just shouted, "Medicine line," and out of the day room, out of the long hallway and off to the exercising porch, body-twisted men shuffle their way forward and form a line just outside the door of the medicine room.

They are distorted in body and face, every one of them, but they are not insane. They are the victims of encephalitis, or sleeping sickness.

Before I was committed here, if I thought of sleeping sickness at all, I thought of it as some vague malady limited to South Africa and induced by the bite of the tsetse fly or some other insect. My shadowy idea was badly wrong. Now I know that in every city of any considerable size, and in some small towns and on farms there are unhappy victims physically distorted by the sequelae or after-effects of this disease. The better physicians know it, and those who are honest admit that medical science has learned but little about how to combat the malady, and less about how to overcome its after-effects.

But the physicians at this hospital are carrying out a series of experiments which, so far, seem to offer a distinct ray of hope for the eventual cure of these terrible effects. And these experiments are the reason why a line of "limber-necks," as the patients call them, forms at the door of the medicine room twice each day. Practically all the encephalitis victims in the institution have been gathered recently into this ward to undergo the long treatment. And what a different looking set of men it is which now faces the charge attendant from the one which shuffled past him when the sufferers were first brought to the ward.

Whether the new treatment will result in permanent cures remains to be seen, but it is unquestionably true that it makes startling improvement in the patients while it is being administered.

Physicians everywhere are watching the results. A vast field of human suffering may be overcome through knowledge acquired here.

When they began taking the treatment several of the patients had their heads drawn backward so far that they were forced to look straight upward all the time. The upper lips of most of them were drawn upward in a continual snarl; hands, arms and legs were twisted or feet turned to one side. One or two had their heads drawn down on one shoulder. Most of them could not feed, dress or otherwise care for themselves.

Now all who have been taking the treatment can feed, dress and care for themselves, their heads have straightened up or come forward, limbs and feet have improved, and nearly all of them are very helpful around the ward. To my untrained eye several of them appear to be about ready to go out and resume a place in the world. But this would be extremely bad judgment. It is far better to have them remain here for a time in order that the physicians may study the effects after the medicinal treatment is stopped. It may be that the good effects are but temporary.

Even the physicians who incline to this view say that the treatment marks a distinct advance in overcoming the effects of encephalitis, because it is decidedly inexpensive and a patient could have the medicine administered by his family doctor, whenever it again became necessary.

Atropine sulfate, very poisonous in ordinary amounts, is the basis of the treatment. A few drops of a weak solution of it are administered at the start. Each day the dose is increased by one drop. This is continued until the maximum dosage which it is believed the patient can stand is reached. Then the doses are decreased by one drop each day until the original amount is reached. The treatment is then discontinued and the patient carefully observed. If conditions warrant it the course is repeated.

The patients who were used in the experiments here all showed remarkable improvement within a few days. And the happiness of most of them was almost pathetic.

They were, I imagine, like blind men would be if they were suddenly given a sight of the great world, and the possibility was held out to them that they might gain perfect sight after a time.

One of the patients is a young man for whom I write letters. He has never learned to read or write as he has been afflicted since early childhood. He could hold nothing in his hands, and his head was drawn back so far that he could not see where he was walking. He could not feed himself.

Now his letters to his father bubble with his hope that soon he will be coming home, cured. We try to keep him from becoming too enthusiastic; we are afraid that the disappointment would be too bitter if the improvement should prove to be only temporary. But his exuberant happiness refuses to consider any such possibility.

He sweeps and polishes floors, helps to carry meals to those who are in bed, and does other ward tasks as well as any of the patients. But his greatest thrill came the other day on the baseball grounds. He was permitted to take a small part in a practice game. He knew nothing about it: he has never played. But he could run bases for the batters: actually run, when only a month or so ago his halting walk was a directionless, dragging shuffle. No wonder he was nearly hysterically happy.

The assistant superintendent of the hospital, the same physician who has been so thoughtful of me, is the man who developed and is carrying out the experimental treatment. He has made it almost a game for the victims of the malady. Daily he would line the distorted fellows up like a bunch of raw army recruits and put them through a series of physical movements designed to test their improvement.

He had them bend and try to touch their hands to the floor, wheel at command, walk a straight line, go through simple calisthenics and otherwise attempt voluntary use of their muscles. Their efforts were pitiful at first, but what good progress they made! Even the worst distorted of them now is straightened into a practically normal position.

Speed the good work!

In the past the other patients have not liked these limber-necks, most of whom have been helpless for a long time. They have had to be waited upon—by members of their families before they came here; by patients since they reached this hospital. And waiting on a limber-neck was an unpleasant task. They had always been humored and "babied" by the members of their families and they were not slow to find fault, nastily, when they were not babied after their arrival here.

But with their physical improvement they seem to have recovered from much of their whining expectation of being unduly considered. They have a new mental attitude. They are learning to do their part in life and to be glad to do it. And that is worth as much to them as their physical improvement.

Even though the carefully worked out experiment should accomplish nothing more for other sufferers from encephalitis than it has already done for the men here it has added measurably to human happiness. This is my mead of tribute to the physician who, while taking care of about 350 other patients, yet finds time to devote to thoughtful efforts toward learning new ways for permanently benefiting a great class of unfortunates.

Not that all hospital physicians have such qualities; far, far from it. Attendants have many a chuckle at the expense of some physicians under whom they have worked, and scores of patients have a deep and abiding hatred for some of the physicians who have been connected with this hospital in the past.

An attendant tells of a young physician, not long out of the university, who came, as a ward physician, to an insane hospital.

"I don't believe that bird had ever been near an insane man before, but he knew all about insane people," the attendant told me. "I know he knew all about them because he admitted that he did. Why he knew so much about them that he could tell you just by looking them over whether they were ready to be sent home or not. The very first time he came on the ward he picked out four or five fellows and told me they were ready to go home. The fun of it was that three of them were about the most violent on the ward when they had their disturbed spells. They just happened to be in a rational condition at that time.

"But that young chump thought that if they looked intelligent and talked rationally they were perfectly sane. He phoned me, one day, to let a certain patient go down to the reception room, without an attendant with him, when he had visitors. When they caught that patient he was two hundred miles from the hospital; he had stolen a car to get away in.

"But one of the attendants just about cured him of knowing so much. One of the patients on his ward who was usually quiet had a bad spell one day and the attendant locked him up. When the doctor came through the ward he discovered that the patient was locked in his room and demanded to know why this had been done. The attendant told him the patient was in a dangerous frame of mind, but the doctor thought he knew all about that patient because he had talked to him several times. He ordered the attendant to unlock the door at once. The attendant did so and the patient came charging out in a fighting frenzy and the first man he landed on was that young doctor. The attendant and other patients finally pulled him off but I guess they did not hurry very much about it, and the doctor got pretty well mauled.

"Say! After that, Mr. Know-it-all knew a lot less about who was crazy and who was not."

The "bum" attendants who manage to catch on here for a time tell blood curdling stories about the treatment of patients in some other hospitals. Knowing the character of the men telling the stories I usually add a liberal pinch of salt to the tales before swallowing them. But I believe some of the things they tell do occur, probably at their own hands.

"Say, the guys at this hospital baby these nuts too much," one such attendant told me. "Why at the I —— State hospital some nut got wet-toweled or soaped almost every day. And you can bet those bugs knew better than to talk back."

I know what wet-toweling and soaping mean. Attendants and other patients have told me. Both practices are said to have been very common twenty years ago, and still do persist in practically all hospitals. But now they are used only under conditions of urgent emergency, and are usually prohibited by the hospital management.

Both are sternly prohibited here, but I would not be greatly surprised if some attendant, in a desperate fight, should revert to former training, especially if he believed he could avoid detection. Patients are sometimes afraid to report such cases.

Wet-toweling a patient is choking him unconscious by getting a wet towel around his neck and twisting on it from the back until he succumbs. Sometimes a pillowslip is used instead of a towel. "A wet towel is best," an attendant told me. I did not ask him how he knew what was "best." I had looked him over.

"Before they become unconscious their tongues stick out of their mouths and their eyes bulge out. God, it's awful," one of the patients tells me.

He has never seen any one choked unconscious here, he says, although he has been here many years. But formerly he was confined in a hospital in an Atlantic coast state. "Why I saw an attendant choke an epileptic unconscious and just get up and leave him there on the floor. And he made the rest of us leave him alone; wouldn't let us help the man. After awhile the epileptic began to get his breath and finally got up. I reported that ease and the attendant got fired but the other attendants made me wish I hadn't told," he says.

I do not know how much of this man's story to believe. He is very irrational at times. But I do know that similar cases have occurred. Older attendants have told me that such cases were fairly common until about fifteen years ago, "when the people began to get wise to it." Thank Heaven, even the slow and uninformed indignation of the public sometimes has a good effect.

"Soaping a man down," means knocking him down with a slug made of a hard bar of soap in the toe of a sock. Such a slug will knock a patient down, often rendering him unconscious, without leaving telltale marks. The wet towel treatment also leaves no marks or scars for inquisitive officials, hospital authorities or unexpected visitors to find. Hurrah for the inventive genius of younger America. It finds ways to make itself safe. Of course when it comes to a question of veracity between an attendant and a patient the attendant has a distinct advantage. He has never been declared insane.

Yet when the public does become aroused, through some flagrant ease of brutality that comes to newspaper notice, its blows at the evil conditions are aimed blindly, through its ignorance of the insane and the best methods of handling them. Often these blows are more hurtful than helpful. In some cases they are ridiculous.

In that same state of I———, where, according to the bum attendant's story, soaping and wet-toweling are so common, the state legislature recently passed a law prohibiting the use of strait-jackets on patients. That law is distinctly bad; so bad that it should be repealed immediately, before it results in further injury to patients who can not help themselves.

Its proponents argued that the strait-jacket is brutal; that struggling patients should be restrained only by the hands of the attendants. I am convinced that they never had seen a modern strait-jacket, and it is absolutely certain that they knew nothing of the mental element in the control of patients in a paroxysm, and did not take into consideration conditions existing in every hospital for the insane, under present methods.

A struggling patient will fight to the last atom of his strength when he is being held by human beings. He believes that those holding him are either tempting to hurt him or are enemies. Their very presence stirs his crazed mind to resistance. And the frenzy will continue as long as the men hold him.

Put the same patient into a strait-jacket, tie him to his bed with broad bands of heavy canvas or bed ticking which can not cut or hurt him, and often he will stop struggling very soon. There is no provocative presence of men, opposing their wills to his. He realizes that he is helpless and ceases to fight.

This is but one of the reasons why the law is distinctly a step backward. In this ward, the best in the institution, I have seen as many as three patients tied in bed at one time. They were in a paroxysm and had to be restrained to prevent their injuring themselves or others. If a man attempted to hold them it would require at least four men to each patient, or twelve men where three patients were suffering disturbances simultaneously.

There are never more than three attendants on this ward at any one time. It is seldom indeed that more than two attendants are stationed on any ward. Legislatures which pass foolish measures like the strait-jacket law never increase the appropriations for the hospitals so as to make it possible for them to double the number of attendants and thus be able to comply with the law. No indeed. That would require public money. What would the taxpayers say?

So they just pass a law prohibiting the use of strait-jackets and let the hospital physicians and attendants evolve ways and means. The physicians and attendants, perforce, do just that, and the patients suffer.

In many cases paroxysms last all day and all night and frequently through several days. If the intent of the law were fulfilled several men would be forced to hold the struggling patient every hour of the day and night, their very presence exciting him to resist. Perhaps his heart would fail under the strain or he would burst a blood vessel. Such cases have occurred.

And what of the men who were compelled to restrain him? Attendants could not do it. There are never enough of them. Even if enough shifts of trustworthy patients could be gathered for the purpose the mental reaction on them would be very bad. Such a task should never be imposed on patients. The paroxysms of the fighting patient would have a bad effect on their nervous systems which might throw some of them into a paroxysm, not to mention the wearing and exhausting physical exertion of restraining the patient for hours at a stretch.

So attendants fall back on several methods of restraining patients, any one of which is more harmful and less humane than the use of a properly made strait-jacket. Perhaps the patient may be bound with ropes or straps which may cut or wear into the flesh. Perhaps he may be "packed."

This is the favorite method of evading the law. The patient is tightly wrapped, from head to foot, in heavy sheets, each additional sheet being drawn as tightly as possible. This binds his arms against his sides and prevents use of his legs. Sometimes he even can not move his feet. Circulation is hindered. His sanitary functions cannot be taken care of; he must lie in his own filth until the paroxysm is ended and attendants can unwind his wrappings and give him a bath.

Packing a man does to him just what the uninformed strait-jacket law was intended to prevent. The use of the jacket is far more humane. The patient's arms and hands are enclosed in heavy canvas sleeves which prevent his causing injury but do not hinder circulation. The jacket comes only to the waist and sanitation can be better attended to. In a "pack" he is trussed up worse than if the discarded strait-jackets of twenty years ago were used. But the attendants have broken no law. The sheets and blankets of the pack are not a strait-jacket.

Ho! hum! They say the world is growing better. I wonder if it is also growing wiser. If so, then really informed laws may yet result from the present and growing tendency to pass half considered laws, then go home and consider the matter settled, without any regard for practicality, without proper safeguards being thrown around the selection of the individuals who must enforce those laws, or any proper, well-informed and adequately financed means for bringing about respect for the laws, which is the only basis of full law enforcement.

"Constant breaking of one law creates disrespect for all law." Where have I heard that? Oh, yes, in connection with prohibition. The Volstead law is nominally in force, yet the number of men, women and girls who are sent to various institutions with alcohol-grooved minds is constantly increasing.

I am preaching homilies again. Me and Solomon! What a pair! So far as I know Solomon was never adjudged insane, but I am confident he must have had disturbed spells. One wife and one sweetheart are disturbing enough, but I am told that Solomon did not stop at that.

Even one lady friend can be distinctly disturbing. There is Constance, who continues to send me letters and packages—welcome packages—when I am trying to persuade her not to do so.

The longer I stay here the more I realize that motives and actions inside the state hospitals are quite like those on the outside; just more accentuated and less restrained. The shrewder ones in here manage to get the best of things; those less shrewd are compelled to put up with what they can get. Even in insane asylums the "smart" men best those less calculating. It will always be thus; anywhere.

There is even "grafting" within the wails—and all the stage settings for a racket or two. However I feel sure that it would not pay Al Capone to open a branch office here.

The grafting is limited to getting extra supplies of tobacco, better things to eat and better clothing than other patients. The rackets are worked in the usual way, trading protection or personal services for merchandise.

Some of the patients, who are mentally capable, are put to work in the hospital store. In spite of close watching they manage to carry back to the ward such things as tobacco, snuff, matches, and even breakfast food. These purloined articles serve as the beginning of a chain. The fellow who works in the laundry is glad to take extra pains in seeing that the clothes of a man who works in the store are most carefully washed and returned to the proper owner. He expects a can of smoking tobacco in return. The fellow working in the bakery is willing to filch a few cookies to trade for a plug of tobacco or some raisins or sugar. So the chain goes.

Of course the fellows get caught sometimes. But what of that? How are you to punish a fellow who is already locked up, perhaps for life? As for the moral aspect of it, most insane people have absolutely no moral perception. Some forms of insanity seem completely to erase all conception of right and wrong. If the patients so affected refrain from doing certain things it is not that they realize these things are wrong; it is that they are afraid to do them.

Of course people on the outside are never deterred from doing things through fear; particularly those who preach the punishment of mankind in hell fire.

Nor is the petty grafting entirely confined to the patients. It is only that the patients are more prone to it. They feel that they are outwitting the authorities, and there is a zest in that which is almost as interesting as the things acquired. You see insane people enjoy the feeling of "being able to get away with it."

One man here, with whom I was rather friendly, was put to work keeping records and issuing supplies at the hospital store. For a time he lived high. He had steak with his meals; pies and cakes frequently. Before he was paroled home he managed to acquire two new suits of clothes, two pairs of new shoes, and even some toilet accessories.

It was easy, he boasted. He slipped tobacco, canned goods and other things to the baker and butcher, and received favors in return. He had an ingenious method of getting new clothes and sending them home for his use later on. He had charge of the issuance of clothing, and kept the records, which made getting hold of the articles easy. He acquired the first suit and pair of shoes openly, as the hospital furnishes "Sunday clothing" to the patients. Then he had a brother come to visit him—at the store. The brother slipped the new suit and shoes out and took them home. Later this was repeated.

The trick could not have been worked had the brother been compelled to visit him on the ward. The young man was recently paroled home, and had plenty of clothing to last him for some time.

Of course he could not have got away with so much if he had not prepared the way by trading little favors with susceptible employees. He had issued extra gasoline to several of them and supplied others with goods of various kinds. How could they expose him without exposing themselves? He was quite a business man, in his way. I expect to see him a leader in his community before very long.

I could not expose him. You see he managed to slip me one of those new suits. It is far too large for me. I can not use it. I did not ask for it; he simply slipped into my room with it one night. But I let the suit stay in my room. After that he knew I could not tell on him and he often boasted to me how he was "putting it over" on the physicians.

I still have the suit of clothes, although I have no use for it. Some people hate to give up anything they have acquired free, even if they can not use it.

But the weirdest "graft" is that which centers around the "dead clothes boxes." Patients who die often leave good articles of clothing—a shirt or two, a tie, or good socks. If no relatives claim their things these remain in the "box" where they have been stored during the lifetime of the deceased patient, but not for long. A good shirt or tie soon finds its way to some of the other patients or to an attendant; quite often to an attendant. One of the relief attendants here told me that he had not been compelled to buy a shirt for more than a year. He had not been here long at that time, and now is probably at work in some other hospital. At least he is gone from here.

Some of the patients say that those patients who work in the laundry and some itinerant attendants do not always wait for a patient to die. They claim that shirts and socks are sometimes deliberately "lifted" in the laundry and the owner does not see them again. One patient claims to have lost a shirt and later seen an attendant wearing it. Knowing this particular patient and knowing the strictness of the rules against such things I doubt the story.

But formerly there was a patient here who did steal consistently from other patients. He was the young man who "played crazy" in the penitentiary in order to get transferred to the hospital, and who later was released through the political influence of friends of his father. He was mentally keen and was placed in charge of the room where the clothing of incoming patients is stored in "boxes," arranged like large pigeon-holes around the walls of a room. Each box is labeled with the name of the owner of the articles and a record is kept of everything received.

Several patients complained that articles of good clothing which they had brought in with them were never returned to them. The young man scoffed and pointed to his records of clothing received, to prove that the missing articles were not brought into the hospital. But when he was discharged, suddenly, he did not have time to gather up all of his own belongings; and shirts, shoes and ties which had disappeared were found in his room.

This young man was the one on whom the other patients placed verbal bets that he would be back in the penitentiary before long. Less than three months after he was discharged from the hospital he stabbed a man to death in my home city. In spite of his past record he escaped punishment through a plea of self defense. He will probably kill some one else. He is that kind.

Another of our "sane insane" has left us. He is the fellow whose family was so expensive that he overstepped the law in selling mortgaged property. It happened that the man he defrauded had influence. In some way he managed to have the real estate seller pronounced sane (he was). Then the sheriff took him back to stand trial. The insanity dodge is good—if the other fellow has not too long an arm. Political influence sometimes can accomplish a cure of such "insanity."

I should have neglected civic affairs, and taken up politics.

Such things as the operation of political influence, petty graft, the imposition of the stronger on the weaker and the trading of favors for silence will always exist, as long as human nature is what it is. I can't blame the fellows in the asylum. They learned it outside. And they must look out for themselves. No one comes forward to assist the insane.

Will some one please page our great philanthropists who are giving millions toward founding libraries named for themselves, building fraternity houses at their alma mater, or donating community halls to the towns of their birth, and ask them if the saving of Joan and thousands like her could not be considered as compatible with genuine humanitarian instincts and worth the thought and cash of those who really desire to serve mankind? The message should not be delivered to those who try to buy public approbation like a hot cross bun. They would not understand it.

There is Ted, a young man here, who would make an excellent subject for the first rehabilitation efforts of any kindly soul. He came here suffering from the effects of sleeping sickness. His father was dead, his mother young and attractive.

He has been here several years. The atropine treatment apparently has cured his distorted arm. He is above average intelligence for a youth who has had so little school training. I write his letters for him. He dictates a clear, concise and forceful letter. He is trusted with several minor responsibilities and carries them out with efficiency.

He could make good outside.

But his mother has married again. She does not want her new husband to know that she has a son in the insane asylum. She never writes to the boy. She has moved, and has never let him know her new address. He has been unable to secure it. There is no one to apply for a parole for him.

So he must stay here, youthful energy and ambition burning him cruelly. He apparently is perfectly sane; but legally he is insane, and it may be that he must spend much of his life within the walls of an insane asylum. Is he to blame? Who extends a hand?

Carry on, Ted. Grimly set your jaw and carry on. When you think of life sweeping by on the outside; when that young man's yearning to be accomplishing something sears you, when thoughts of a home, wife, family and friends, torture you; grip your sanity hard, Ted. Don't let go of that. Don't let the life here get you. Perhaps a way may develop.

Who extends a hand?

CHAPTER XI

INTROSPECTION

WE had blackberries and a tiny bit of cake for supper, last night. And we had eggs and biscuits and syrup for breakfast this morning. Two feasts within a thirteen hour period. Yes, thirteen hours elapse between supper and breakfast.

The men could not understand their good fortune, but this did not prevent them from cleaning up everything in sight. They fell to it with a gusto and a mighty clattering that made the attendant in charge of the dining room roar, "Quiet there, you rummies. Where do you think you are, anyhow?"

And Nelson, the irrepressible, who sits at my table and is an alcoholic like myself, leaned over to me and whispered, "We know where we are, all right. We are in a G—— d—— bughouse."

The attendants are at a marked disadvantage in expressing their opinion of the patients. They are not permitted to use profanity or obscenity, and it cramps the vocabulary of some of them woefully. The patients are also prohibited from using profanity, but sometimes they take a chance and do it. They can not be discharged for it as the attendants can—they are already locked in.

The two feasts were doubly welcome. Our fare has been both drab and scanty lately. It is near the end of the fiscal year and I suspect that the steward is making an effort to stay within the budget.

The patients simply can not conjure up any sympathy for the budget. They know only that the food has been scanty, and they growl about it. But they don't do anything about the matter. Convicts sometimes join together and stage a protest when food is scanty, but insane patients never do. They can not cooperate. Their grumbling is all done individually, and to themselves.

Perhaps that is just another indication that they were sent to the right place when they were committed to an insane asylum.

For me there are several reasons why today should be cheerful and noteworthy in addition to the two good meals. There are flowers in my room. I have just received a big package of fruit and cakes. It is Airplane day, and another patient cleaned up my room for me this morning, in return for my writing several letters for him. It's a pretty good world, after all.

The flowers were brought to me by a patient who works in the hospital greenhouse. I have written some letters for him, also, and in here every favor must scrupulously be repaid in some way. The favored patient feels that he is under obligations to you and he can not be comfortable until he has done something for you in return. He will insist on doing something for you, even if it is something you don't want done. Then he feels that responsibility has been lifted from his shoulders. He is care-free again.

As for the airplane, it is a big commercial passenger ship which flies over the hospital three times weekly, plying between two cities. It is a source of excitement here on every trip. Many of the patients have been here for years and never saw an airplane except this one. They have never seen this ship except in the air, but they like to watch it and wonderingly speculate about it. Their conception of what makes it go and how it is guided and handled is vague and fantastic. But there is a big rush for the exercising porch when its motor is heard. It offers some break in the monotony. And I, the holder of a private pilot's license, find my feet leading me to the porch also.

The package of edibles? It is just one of many sent me by Constance, my "lady friend" back in my home city. Constance—in the old days just a Light o' Love; not even a passing flame.

Just one of the various women who shared my wild parties with me, and became as loving and possessive as most women do on wild parties.

But then, with something of a shock, I discovered that she was just as loving and possessive with me when she was cold sober, and that was the very last thing in the world that I wanted. I wanted no woman in the universe to have any claim on me, or any interest in me, except as a partner on a carousal. Party women, just party women, that is all I wanted; just the kind of women who love, and forget next morning; and then look for another party.

So I cut that affair off short. Frankly, almost brutally, I told her why. I was completely free and determined to remain so. Besides she just was not my kind. No more parties with her, for me. And no dates of any kind. I was through.

But was I? She pleaded that she was a "good sport," admitted that she was infatuated with me, but swore by all the gods there may be that at any time I wanted her to let me go my way she would do so without a murmur or protest. And, she argued, whenever I was looking for a good time why not include her in it? Why deprive her of pleasure? She would understand; she promised, she swore it.

Perhaps she thought she meant it. But she did not. She either would not or could not leave me alone. I told her, time and time again, brutally, that I did not love her, could not love her; could never love her. I would refuse to see her for weeks at a time, return her letters unopened, refuse to answer her telephone calls. She would send some friend to me begging that I see her, or send me a letter by messenger boy, instructing him not to come back without an answer. She tried everything from hysteria to pretended serious sickness to draw me to her.

And I reacted just as the average man does under such circumstances. With a normal man the more frantically a woman pursues him the more frantically he flees. I was learning that when a highly emotional woman becomes infatuated with a man his only escape is in leaving the state—and hiding his trail so that it can not be unearthed.

But whenever my continual drinking reached one of its climaxes in a several weeks' sodden debauch, putting me in a hospital, weak, ill and nerve racked, it was she who sent me flowers, flew to the hospital, remained at my bedside every moment that the hospital authorities would permit her to be there, watched over me like a mother over a feverish child—and nursed me back to health.

And in those tortured hours of physical weakness and mental let-down, when the fibers of will and resistance were dissolved and I needed the strengthening touch of some one, just any one, who cared, I was grateful to have her near. And she knew this, in spite of my harsh denials and my ungracious protests at her presence.

It was she who saved my life in that last terrible experience which brought me here. Raving on the brink of delirium tremens from a debauch which had continued for weeks, I had called a physician to try to bring me back to sobriety and health. I happened to call a Doctor Pomposity Nincompoop; one of those physicians, and their name is legion, who know nothing about how to treat alcoholic cases or how to handle men in the madness of whiskey delirium, but who accept the cases nevertheless, and sometimes permanently injure body or brain, or even kill men.

He had me locked up in a hotel room, and abruptly shut off my supply of liquor. I must not have another drop, he instructed the hotel management.

He dosed me with paraldehyde, a hypnotic designed to drug the victim to sleep, and topped this with a furious dose of a bromide solution.

Then, humming gaily to himself, he went away, leaving me crazed out of all conscious knowledge, locked in a room with no water, no whiskey, no one to look after me—and eight ounces of paraldehyde and a pint bottle of bromide solution in plain sight on the bureau.

Some time during the mad delirium of the next forty-eight hours, throughout which I raved and shrieked for water, for whiskey, I managed to reach the bureau and take both of those bottles back to bed with me. I have no recollection of doing it, but in some way I did it. The twin devils of screaming thirst and demoniacal mental torture were riding me; the fluid in those bottles must have mocked me. I may have thought it was water. Or I may have thought it was whiskey. At least it was something which could be drunk. So I drank it.

Certain it is that when Constance found me I was drinking the last of the paraldehyde and bromide solution, though scarcely able to raise my arms or my head from the bed, and in my distorted imaginings I was fighting fiendish, gibbering creatures which even a case of delirium tremens could not conjure up unaided.

It was the whiskey, paraldehyde and bromide mixed, abetted by physical weakness, which was doing that.

Something psychic in her make-up must have called her to me and enabled her to find me. She felt that something was wrong with me. She 'phoned to my newspaper and found that I was "reported sick," a common occurrence in my case. The managing editor and city editor knew what caused these illnesses, but they kept me on the payroll.

If anyone expressed surprise at this the managing editor shrugged his shoulders and replied that if I were drunk half the time I could do more and better work than many men who stayed sober seven days in the week.

But that psychic something told her that I was in serious trouble. How she managed to locate me I will never know. Not one of my friends or acquaintances knew where that doctor had left me. They did not know the doctor. I had never called him before. I did not know who I was calling when I 'phoned him. With my mind in the first grip of delirium tremens I had brushed the phantasmal fiends from before me with shaking hands, staggered to the telephone and called the first physician on whose telephone number I could focus my reeling eyes. He had left me at a hotel where I was not known. But she found me.

Her means are slender—a tiny income left her by her husband who obligingly died ten years ago. But she called an ambulance, hurried me to a good hospital, guaranteed the bills, and hovered over me day and night, while physicians and nurses fought to keep me from passing over the brink.

For two weeks they expected me to die almost any minute. Could that faint spark be kept burning? The doctors did not know; no one knew. Yet even as they thought they were losing, the doctors fought on, spurred by her entreaties and her frantic hope. Intravenous injections, spinal injections, the last desperate calls to that flickering life spark were tried.

As for me, those two weeks are gone out of my life. It is as though they never had been. Then came the turn; not to consciousness at first, but to wild hallucinations as the triple drugs began to let go their hold, to unrealities that no sane mind could reach, yet experiences so real to me that to this day, long months afterward, I am not able to separate the actual events from the drug-conjured ones.

And during that delirium she sat by my bed. Doctors and nurses could not drive her away. They found that I could be quieted better by her touch than in any other way. She would slip off to another room, cry her heart out, dry her eyes and resume her place at my bedside. She has told me, since, that while I was delirious I always called her "Sweetheart." She cries yet, when she tells me that.

She located my relatives; telephoned them. But something had died in them. They had helped me through so many of my derelictions, had come to my rescue such numberless, fruitless times. So they sent—sympathy. She fought on unaided.

My mind dragged but slowly from under the clouds. I could not think rationally. I could not even consider my own case. My body hesitatingly, haltingly grew stronger, but my nervous system shivered brokenly.

I could not control my shaking hand sufficiently to sign my name. I could not think in sequence. The physicians ascribed that to "bromide intoxication, with complications." There was some talk of "giving the facts to the County Medical Association" and letting that body consider Doctor Nincompoop's case. Of course it was never done. No physician was willing to take the lead. It might bring reprisals on his head.

The hospital authorities began to grow restive about their bills. I had spent thousands of dollars on "liquor cures" and hospitals, all to the credit of Booze, within the last few years, and I was down nearly to my last cent.

She could make only small payments on the big bill. She took me to her own hotel room; cared for me, fed me and nursed me back to sanity, but sanity of a weary, pitiful sort.

Then she rallied my friends. They were for me, but they wanted to see me cured of the liquor habit.

They held earnest counsel. They decided that the only way to save me—what was left of—was to confine me for a long period where it was impossible for me to get whiskey, but where I could get medical supervision, of a kind. They had me declared insane. Some of my close friends sat on the lunacy board. The judge who committed me had previously written me several letters gratefully thanking me for my editorial support of him in his campaign for election.

As for me, I did not care. I could not care. My mind was not in a condition to think, to visualize. It was immovably heavy, out of function, deadly weary. I knew only that I wanted to be cured of my desire for whiskey, and to have time to recover, to get strong, in body and mind.

So they sent me here. She came with me when the deputy sheriff brought me. She turned back, crying, when they started to lead me to the receiving ward, so she never heard the key grate when the door was locked behind me.

She has sent me everything she could think of to make my lot more endurable; has done it in spite of my letters begging her not to do so. Magazines, fruit, cake, candy, ribbons and paper for my typewriter—a score of little things which only a woman would think of. I write and scold her for doing so, when I know that she is depriving herself in order to buy things for me. Back comes a tearful letter telling me that it makes her happy to do things for me, and I must not scold her for doing what she enjoys.

Did I say Light o' Love?' What manner of man am I?

And yet, ——

I think of her stormy jealousies, her bitter and unrestrained tongue when she is aroused, her lack of inborn refinement, her glaring clothes and garish manners.

I think of how her nature rasps mine, of how she could not long stand my characteristics and I could never learn to endure hers. I picture the inevitable and endless bitter recriminations which would make up our lives if we should attempt to live together. We have nothing in common, and a thousand clashing characteristics.

When I "go home" I have the world to whip, and I must start from back of taw, at middle age. Either my background will be inescapably tarnished or I must go to some city where I am not known and start without a background; without a revealable past. In either case such a woman would not only make both of us eternally miserable, but would constitute an almost unconquerable handicap in the race for standing and substance.

It is not alone that she is of common strain but that mingled with this are traces of coarseness, visible to any observer, displeasing to the more fastidious. I could not take her to the country club, a banquet or any theater party where I might meet friends. She is not that kind.

She would not let me go alone. She is not that kind.

Yet it is at such places that acquaintance, standing, influence and profit are built in these gilded days.

I know that she is madly determined that I shall marry her as soon as I get my final parole. If there is any one in the world to whom I owe an undischargeable debt she is the one. Would such a union, even though she wishes it, be discharging the debt, or merely assuring misery to us both?

Curiously her name is Constance.

Constance, you and fate and my multiple follies have conspired to put the hardest problem of my life squarely up to me.

Which way out?

CHAPTER XII

THE HALTING ADVANCE

WILD BILL got into trouble with one of the attendants yesterday, and today he did not come down to breakfast or dinner. Wild Bill was ashamed, and sulking.

I do not know his real name and I believe that not half a dozen of the patients know him by any name other than Wild Bill. But every patient, old and new, knows him by that title. It would be impossible to be here long and not know him.

For one thing he has the only well developed, drooping mustache on the ward. For another, well there is no other patient just like Wild Bill.

He is a rather small, well set-up man, as quick on his feet as a cat. In his youth he was a prize-fighter; the sort of prize fighter who depends on his hands and not his head. He could not have used his head to any advantage. He has the mental development and characteristics of a boy of ten years, who is below average intelligence.

Some of the other patients say that he is "punch nutty;" that he is here because his head stopped too many hard packed gloves flung at him by fighters who mixed some thinking with their footwork and slugging. I doubt it. A person, even a prize fighter, must once have had some brains in order to have been knocked crazy.

Bill is eternally and continually directing rough horseplay at the other patients, whacking them lustily on the back when they least expect it, tripping them up without warning, and such little pleasantries. But he flies into a temper if anyone tries the same games on him. His flashes of temper last about three seconds, on the average, but it takes him only a fraction of that time to shoot a still powerful wallop at the offender, and by the time he becomes sorry for his outburst the other fellow may be wearing a swelled jaw or decorated eye.

Of course no "practical joker" on the outside ever becomes angry at being on the receiving end of the rough horseplay that he inflicts on others. But then, you see, Bill has the mentality of a ten year old child.

If he discovers that any of the other patients are ticklish he makes life miserable for the fellow with the sensitive ribs. His tickling is apt to have all the gentleness of the rake of a grizzly bear's claws, when the grizzly is not fooling.

But yesterday Bill made the mistake of trying his ticklish stunt on an attendant. The attendant retaliated by giving Bill himself a rib-torturing tickling, and Bill is about the most ticklish person I ever saw. He writhed and shrieked and finally squirmed loose, in a towering temper. He aimed a right swing at the attendant's jaw, but the attendant does not believe in unpreparedness. He hunched a shoulder, after the manner of a good defensive boxer, and took the blow on a well cushioned clavicle. Then he seized Bill and held him helpless until his momentary temper burned out."

Go to that chair and sit down. And stay there until I give you permission to move," he ordered. Bill's jaw dropped. He, Wild Bill, was being punished. He was in disgrace. He was being told to sit in a chair. It was like being made to stand in the corner when he was a child at school.

But Bill's mentality is that of a child. In a moment he was crying, just like a punished child, in spite of his forty-three years and his cherished mustache. He was sorry; he "didn't mean to do it," he told the attendant again and again, while tears ran down his cheeks. The attendant was adamant, although his eyes twinkled when he was not looking at Bill. So Bill was compelled to sit quietly for a half hour before he was forgiven.

But he felt the disgrace. He did not come down to breakfast or to dinner. "Leave him alone," the attendant ordered when some of the other patients tried to persuade Bill to go down to dinner. "He will go when he gets hungry enough."

And Bill did. Tonight he came shamefacedly to his supper. And how he did eat. His penitence will be as short lived as his flashes of temper. Tomorrow he will be full of crude horse play again.

I missed Bill, gratefully, while he was sulking in his self-punishment. He eats at my table. And I do not relish his kind of horseplay. For some reason I dislike to have pieces of bread thrust down the back of my neck whenever I turn my head to see what the fellow on the other side of me is doing.

We are seated four to a table, and each quartet is selected with care. I am at the same table with Bill to act as a steadying influence on him and another patient who sits just across from me. This young fellow is what is termed a "silly" by the other patients. He is not insane, in the usual acceptation of the word. He is given to silly grimaces, silly remarks, silly caprices. He is just a "silly."

Many youths have a temporary period of silliness just as they are changing from boyhood into manhood, but with this young man the silliness did not disappear. It became permanent. Members of his family, cultured people, were embarrassed continually by his silliness in the presence of other people and his morbid and unrestrained interest in anything of the feminine sex. They had him committed here.

They keep him supplied with pocket money and bring him fruits, cakes, pies, candies and other enticing edibles whenever they come to visit him. I suppose they feel that they are very kind to him and thoughtful for him. But he is here for life.

His silliness is not at all disturbing to me. His morbid and foolish interest in women is. As he sits at the table he is continually craning his neck to see through the open door into the kitchen, where women work.

Of course none of the men patients are permitted to go in there, but he can see the women, and conjure up thoughts.

"See that one? Look. Look. Right there at that table. She looked at me. She's looked at me twice. Wait a minute. Maybe she'll do it again." He smirks and continues to crane his neck.

The woman may be forty, fat and frowsy. But she is a woman, and he is sillily interested.

But, wait a minute. I am middle aged and he is but twenty-six. It might be possible that at his age I would have craned my neck in order to look at just any sort of woman, and, like him, I might continually have watched the broad concrete walks outside to see if I could spy a woman attendant, passing along.

On second thought, I am not so old. And I am going to get out before so very long. Chuckle, darn you. What are you laughing about?

"Whizbang Mabel" gave Silly a real thrill, recently. She walked right into the dining room and up to his table. And she made coyly provocative remarks.

Just for that little thing Whizbang Mabel is not working in the kitchen, any longer. She is banished to her ward. And Whizbang is dreadfully displeased about it. She voices her displeasure almost every night. When the chorus of screams and shrieks and cries from the women's ward across the court is going full blast Whizbang's mighty voice swings in and the former bedlam is dwarfed; belittled.

No weakling is Whizbang. Five feet, seven inches, and 195 pounds, Mabel stands, in her swearing clothes. Not that she needs any clothes to swear in, but the rules of the institution provide that a woman must have something on besides a tantrum.

At profanity and obscenity Whizbang is a creative artist. Most of her epithets are not copies; they are originals. They are entirely new and unused until she bellows them forth.

In the long distance and hair-raising classes, she is hereby awarded the world's championship in stupendous stultifying.

Mabel is compelled to do her best if she is to retain her titles. She has a talented rival in a scrawny little woman with a high pitched, penetrating voice. The judges, who gather at the barred windows on this side of the court, have conceded the championship to Whizbang owing to her versatility and her wider range; but upon her scrawny rival we have conferred the degrees of Master of Irritating Invective and Professor of Prurient Profanity.

Whizbang's brief elevation to the ranks of kitchen workers, and her subsequent downfall, is a study in elemental human psychology; of the emotions and courses of action which motivated us before civilization laid its inhibitions upon us, and which still do control us when inhibitions have been ingloriously kicked out of the mental penthouse.

Whizbang's obsession is men. Her profanity is not an obsession; it is a combination of safety valve, expression of opinion and high art. Since she believes in forthrightness and directness in her approach to men she was kept closely in her own ward for a time, where the only opportunity she had of seeing men was when they passed along the walks near the windows of her building. Then she would shout shameless advances at them.

But thwarted women sometimes develop cunning. Mabel became good, very, very good. She was a model of dutifulness and propriety. For three or four months her conduct was exemplary, and the authorities were both surprised and pleased. When she asked to be assigned to the kitchen they were willing to give her a trial, especially as she is an excellent and surprisingly tidy cook.

To the kitchen she went, and the first day, with the exception of sly glances through the open door, her conduct was decorum itself. She was considering ways and means.

Some of the fortunate patients, who have the necessary pocket money, are permitted to purchase steaks and other articles of food and have them prepared in the kitchen. Whizbang considered this and saw her golden opportunity.

Silly is one of the men who have steaks cooked in the kitchen. Mabel prepared his steak for him; did it daintily, even to placing it on a bed of lettuce leaves and garnishing it.

Then, having prepared her approach to Silly's heart, through his stomach, she watched her opportunity and when the attendant was not looking she marched straight into the dining room and up to our table, simpering and coy. Possibly she might have got away with this infraction of the rules, but, flushed by the nearness of the men and her success so far, she could not resist going further.

She set the platter down in front of Silly with a flourish. "There you are, Sweetheart," she said. "Didn't I cook it nice for you?" And she gave his hand a provocative pat. She is back on her ward, and nightly she expresses her disappointment, and thwarted love, in outbursts which make some of the lesser performers hush in awed admiration. It was ever thus. A woman thwarted—you know the rest. Oh, tiddle-de-dum.

Silly, with his morbid interest in the other sex, is not a fair example of most of the simple-minded fellows who are here. Several of them have really admirable qualities, aside from their lack of mental development.

There is one "boy" who is one of the most lovable youths I ever met. I wish I might help him in some way. He has developed an embarrassing fondness for me; embarrassing in that he will sit in my room for hours in worshipful silence, much like an adoring dog. And this not only interferes with my work but is apt to cause him to forget his own duties, and thus lose some of his excellent standing with the attendants.

To keep yourself in good standing with the attendants you must not neglect your work, for work is the criterion by which most of the attendants judge all patients. If you are able and willing to do any work assigned you then you may reach the happy state of being classified as "good help on the ward." Otherwise the attendant may tell the physician, "He is of no use to us at all. Send him to some other ward. Maybe that will straighten him out."

Those who are unusually "good help on the ward" have a chance to remain on the receiving ward instead of being transferred to less desirable ones.

Under the state law no patient can be compelled to work. It is a good law. To some degree it protects helpless patients who might happen to be placed under the control of overbearing, slave-driving attendants. Most patients are more than glad to work. It helps to kill the dead monotony. And the attendants can find ways to prod up the lazy and the laggards, such as withholding tobacco rations, keeping them off the baseball field and denying them other privileges; while patients who are too ill or too feeble to work can not be compelled to do so.

Don, the young man who is so exactly like a lovable boy, is an excellent and cheerful worker. He does whatever he is asked to do, in just the way that a dutiful child would. But he has the physique of a healthy young man.

He has the respectful and thoughtful manners of a shy, well raised child. I never met his parents, but I know that at least one of them knows how to raise children. Don got as far as the fourth grade in school, then he developed mysterious headaches, and his mind ceased to grow. But it takes fond parents some time to come to a realization that their child's mind is standing still. Even when they discover the sad fact each will try to conceal it from the other.

When Don's parents did finally acknowledge the facts to themselves they took the boy to good specialists. Every medical attention was given him. But the physicians could not determine the cause of his trouble. So Don's parents sent him to a farm which they owned, hoping against hope that the outdoor exercise and fresh air would snap whatever cord was binding down his mental growth.

When he was about eighteen he suffered a recurrence of those headaches. His mind was blank for a time. Alarmed, his parents sent him here. He recovered and they came and got him and took him back to the farm. Not long ago his mind again went under a cloud. He was hurried back here. He is twenty-one now.

He has come out from under the cloud and again is a shy, sensitive, likable child. But he has reached a man's physical development, and the physicians hold no hope that he will ever fully recover. He has been here several months and his parents have not come for him. I am afraid that they have lost hope of his restoration and believe that it is best for him to remain here. I am not criticizing them. They have their other children to consider. But, oh! what a pity that this likable boy-man must spend the remainder of his life among distorted minds! Considerate of everyone else, with the nicest manners imaginable, not only willing but glad to do anything he is asked to do and always thinking of little things he can do for some one else, he is just a mannerly, well intentioned boy, raised by a good mother.

"Look at him," snorts Lawton indignantly. "As good intentions as any boy that ever walked. Wouldn't do a thing wrong if he lived to be a hundred years old. Yet the state keeps him shut up here with twisted loons. If he stays here long enough he will probably go crazy; as crazy as the rest of them. That is what the states are doing; taking people who are not crazy and locking them up with howling lunatics, to make them go insane. Put the sanest man in the world in here long enough and his mind will crack.

"The world has not yet learned to include peace of mind in the treatment of mental cases," he snorts again and tramples off to his room, with high indignation at the hodge-podge treating of all mental cases alike, fairly oozing from him.

Lawton is an unusually intelligent and well-read man. His thought processes are clear cut and analytical. His reasoning cuts right to the heart of a question, avoiding any clouding issues in any matter except one, and that one is his church. His church is the most profound force in the world; in religion, in politics, in finance, in education, in predicting the rise and fall of nations, in the development of thought and in the final destiny of all mankind.

And yet Lawton is not a religious zealot, in the usual sense. He is too intelligent for that. There is no raving, on his part, about his church, which is one of the oldest in existence. He has no "disturbed spells." He does not attempt to proselytize others to his faith. He really does not intend to intrude his views on others. "I am merely giving you the facts for your information; I know that you do not want to be misinformed," he says after correcting the views of some other man, because they did not coincide with the teachings of his church.

"The church has foreseen this by centuries of time," he is apt to say when listening to a discussion of the World War, the financial depression, the tariff wall around the great trading nations, or the prohibition question. "Not only did The Church foresee it but provided a clear path around it by its action in 1463." He will outline the action taken in 1463, or whatever other date is applicable, and explain how it applies to the question under discussion. "I just don't want you to be misinformed," he says in completely closing the matter. So far as he is concerned the question is completely closed as soon as he has explained the stand of "The Church" on it.

Yes I consider him insane. I do not know what he thinks about my own mental condition. He has been too kind to tell me.

Perhaps I am just not mentally advanced far enough to appreciate the fact that The Church has never made an error, even of omission. He is prone to excuse some of those who disagree with him because they are not mentally advanced enough to comprehend that The Church always has been, and always will be, infallible. He is quite tolerant, kindly so, of those whose minds are not advanced.

In his youth he fell victim to a social disease, and the spirochete, the dread micro-organism of that disease, found its way into his spinal column and thence to his brain. It seems to have affected but the one mental groove in which reposed his religious convictions. Otherwise he is superior to the average intelligent man in reasoning. He was wealthy, well known and popular and, I am convinced, was an admirable man until the spirochete quirked that one part of his brain.

But the quirk grew until it not only distressed but frightened his family and friends. Let the idea that a man is insane once be hinted about him and people will scatter from him like a covey of young quails flushed by a playful collie puppy.

So Lawton came here. He stayed several months, then was discharged and went back to his family. He quickly found that former friends avoided him, shunned him—actually feared him. So he moved his family to a distant state, where no one knew that he had once been committed to an insane asylum. But his family knew.

Whenever there was any difference of opinion between himself and his wife or children there was but one reason in their minds. It was because he was crazy, and was proving that he was crazy by failing to agree with them. So Lawton came back. His family insisted on his doing so; insisted through court action.

They get the benefit of all his property. If he is discharged again, as he hopes to be, he must start all over again, in a new location, without the benefit of a single acquaintance. He seems to be resigned to this.

"My family is provided for," he says. "I have told ambition goodbye. All I desire now is just to make a living of some kind for myself during my remaining years. I believe I can do that. My wants are simple. Since I have been here I have learned just how little a person can get along with."

He and I have discussed the hapless condition of Joan, the girl who dances so well; Don, the young man with the shy mind of a boy, and scores of other patients in this and other state hospitals who may be psychopathic cases but certainly are not insane to the point that they would constitute any sort of menace if set free.

They are not insane, but they can not go back to the outside world without being tagged with the stigma of insanity, in the minds of every one who knows of their past. Once so tagged, and feared, they are shunned or under suspicion, even by their relatives. And how the news is whispered about.

Yet they are entitled to some part of happiness. They should not be locked in with lunatics and subjected to the same rigorous discipline and unending, mind-destroying repression.

Lawton believes he can outline just what is necessary to overcome this palpable injustice.

"I was a fool to think that even my family would understand, after I once had been declared legally insane," he says. "People simply have not advanced far enough for that.

"The final remedy, of course, lies in the proper education of the people to make them understand that every mental case is not insanity. But before that, psychiatrists, broad-minded men and women, and even the leaders in government can accomplish a great deal.

"Psychiatrists who are worthy the name and not just charlatans battening on credulous people, understand fully that scores of people develop a line of thought or a complex which is detrimental to themselves and perhaps to their families and friends, but is not insanity," he points out. "They know also that there are cases of arrested mental development and other mental cases where the victims could not be considered lunatics by any stretch of the imagination. Neurotics are not lunatics. But if they happen to fall into the hands of ignorant relatives or associates, or the average lunacy board, they are very apt to be declared insane and committed to an asylum. That wrecks their entire future, irrevocably.

"Now suppose that each state maintained an observation hospital, separate and distinct from the asylums; situated in a different locality, to which people could be sent without being declared legally insane. They thus would retain their legal standing and control of their affairs until the physicians of the observation hospital had studied them and pronounced them sane or insane.

"Mental cases which should not be sent to an insane asylum could be cared for in the observation hospital, while insane patients could be sent to the regular institutions." He pauses and points out of the window at the row on row of hospital buildings.

"In the big hospitals now maintained, it is impossible for the physicians to give anything but the most cursory attention to any patient. A doctor has just about time enough to dash into a ward, go through it on a run and dash to the next one. He is compelled to look on patients in the mass; he has no time to consider any of them individually or to study their individualities. The system tends to make a cold-blooded machine of a physician, even one with the most conscientious intentions.

"In an observation hospital, where the outflow to the insane asylums and the discharges would keep the number of patients down to a very low point, individual cases could be effectually studied, and the results of such study passed on to the asylums in those cases which require confinement, while those persons who do not require confinement, including paralytics, victims of sleeping sickness and amnesia, aged people and cripples whose families or acquaintances have shunted them into the hospital, could be kept in the observation hospital, avoiding the stigma of legal insanity.

"Right there is where philanthropy should step in. Men and women who now devote their time, thought and money to rehabilitating former convicts would devote a part of their efforts to reestablishing the patients from the observation hospitals, if they could be properly informed and interested. They are afraid to extend aid to those who have been pronounced insane.

"Wealthy men might even build homes to care for such people until they could establish themselves."

When a man or woman, boy or girl, goes out of the present hospitals he or she has not a cent, no clothing to speak of, and no place to go to until employment is secured. If the families of such persons don't want them or if they have no families, what are they going to do? If they are asked for references they can't give them. They are helpless."

Now The Church foresaw this and——" But I hurriedly interrupt.

"The authorities of some hospitals are taking steps in that direction," I remind him. "Some have established observation wards, and they try to separate the patients into classes——"

"Yes," Lawton snorts. "And how do they separate them? I'll tell you. They divide them into good patients and bad patients, regardless of whether they are sane or insane.

"Take this ward. There are men on it who are incurably insane; just as insane as anyone in the entire hospital. They are kept here because they are quiet and have learned to obey orders. But their minds are twisted. They are crazy. Their thoughts are crazy. Keep a sane person cooped up with them long enough and he will go crazy too; especially if he is a neurotic to begin with. Then all of them, even the old men, have to live under rules formulated for the control of lunatics. And they are all legally insane.

"Everyone here has been declared insane. That means that every one is insane in the eyes of the people outside. Think of how my family looked upon me. The fact that I had been here once made it possible for them to send me back. Now The Church ——"

But I fling myself into the breach again.

"The hospital authorities were not responsible for your being declared insane. They did their part when they paroled you as cured."

Lawton's snort is now almost a roar. "Isn't that what I said? Didn't I say that the public must be educated? County judges and fussy old family doctors don't know anything about mental cases, yet they are permitted to declare a man insane and condemn him for life.

"The most they should be permitted to do is to send a patient to the observation hospital where experienced physicians, men who know mental diseases and insanity, to some degree at least, could pass on them after close study extended over a period of time. Now The Church believes in long study of any important question before passing——"

But I gather up my pencil and notes and flee—from The Church.

However Lawton has the germ of the right idea. If only the public could be educated to it sufficiently!

What can anyone do when he is paroled home from here? What can I do and where should I go, when I go home? Will I be asked to head the drives to raise the yearly funds for the chamber of commerce? And will the gentlemen of the Rotary club turn gratefully to me whenever the scheduled speaker fails to show up at the regular weekly luncheon meeting? Will my home city, where I have been a "well known civic worker" for years and where thousands know me, welcome me back with a wholehearted pat on the back, or with a good, hefty kick directed at the widest sector of my trousers?

I can not tell myself a lie. I will need a pair of steel lined pants. Likewise I should undergo an operation for the complete removal of all my sensibilities, feed my pride a lethal dose of cyanide and somehow acquire a grim callousness to slights, slurs and suspicions.

When I go home I will still be legally insane; no patient in this institution is ever actually discharged as cured. He is paroled home and remains under parole for three months, At the end of that time his parole automatically becomes a discharge, But if he should commit any untoward act during that three months the hospital authorities would be protected from possible suits. He is never pronounced sane after he has once been declared insane.

In the meantime how am I to maintain myself. I can not resume control of even the tiny bit of cash remaining to me. If I go to another city where my past is not known I must ask strangers for employment, and then will come the inevitable inquiries as to where I was employed last and the request for references. There will be a long interim which I can not truthfully explain away.

And when prospective employers communicate with the managing editor of the newspaper on which I was last employed is it not common sense to believe that the reply will read:

"In answer to yours of the third inst. will say that Mr.—— was employed by us until a year ago and we found him a valuable man. But I feel that it is my duty to tell you that since that time he has been confined in the state hospital for the insane——"

Oh, well! Perhaps I can put a black patch over one eye and peddle pencils on a street corner.

That brings out another thought. Would Constance be quite so sure that she is anxious to acquire me if she knew that this would entail a step downward, financially and in the estimation of all who might know us? Does she realize what it means to have been adjudged insane?

I am just realizing it, now.

CHAPTER XIII

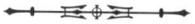

SILHOUETTES

WHEN it rains gloom, it pours. And the last few, torrid summer days have produced a veritable cloud-burst of things conducive to big, black splotches of gloom.

Old Man Simonds, whom I have avoided sedulously ever since I have been in this hospital, managed to waylay me yesterday and pour his troubles into my ear. A woman in one of the women's wards tried to commit suicide, and missed it through a miscalculation. Several of the patients on this ward are having disturbed spells. My chronic enemy, sciatic neuritis, has had me laid by the heels for two weeks and I have been unable to go to the ball games or the park until yesterday. The chorus of shrieks and screams, prayers and profanity, hymns and obscenities, from the women's ward across the court has been continuous and uninterrupted for two days, and men patients in the ward just beneath us and in the Hydro have added to the irritating din.

And then there are my thoughts. Abetted and stirred on by the gloom spots outside my cranium, they have fiendishly slapped me down, kicked me into a pool of depression and jeered at my efforts to rout them.

Old Man Simonds formerly was the editorial writer on the daily newspaper by which I was employed at the time my friends sent me here. He preceded me here by about three years; an incurable paranoiac, the physicians believe.

For seven years we worked on the same newspapers. I knew him intimately. I know his story and I have pieced out his history. I am deeply sorry for him, and that is why I have avoided him ever since I came here. I do not want my feelings harrowed when I cannot help him; when no one can help him.

In the newspaper world he has been widely known for years. He has held important editorial positions on some of the largest newspapers in America. Marital troubles proved the first stumbling block in his career.

I do not know who was to blame. But it was over these troubles that his paranoia later developed. His wife came from an influential and prominent family and Simonds incurred, or thought he had incurred, the enmity of the whole clan. His family life broke up.

His wife married again. But Simonds imagined that her relatives still bore him malice; that, in fact, they pursued him, determined to injure him. He secured a position in a distant city, severed all ties, and finally ceased communicating with anyone who had been familiar with his past life. But still he believed that his former wife's relatives relentlessly pursued him.

A paranoiac lives in a world created by his own quirked mind. His obsessions are as real to him as hard facts which are susceptible of concrete proof. He knows they are true. Argument is unavailing. His mind is grooved in the line of his delusion.

Gradually Simonds' delusion reached the point where it could not be hid. If he passed two strangers talking on the sidewalk he was convinced that they were plotting against him. When he reached a corner he would peer around it before venturing ahead. He would carefully lock himself in the little office where he ground out his daily editorials, before he dared begin work. In every other way he was fully sane and keenly intelligent. Today he is sane and intelligent, except for his besetting obsession.

Finally his fear overcame his caution. He went to the county sheriff and demanded protection. The sheriff protected him by locking him up in a nice steel cell. Until that day he had been writing editorials admired by thousands. The publisher of the paper had known for a year that Simonds was warped on that one matter. But he was a valuable man.

The publisher continued to employ him, but hired a man to accompany him, unobtrusively, day and night. Simonds, through a trick, evaded this guardian when he made his trip to the office of the sheriff.

Of course the sheriff placed Simonds before the lunacy board and he was committed here. He has been here for more than three years. His mind runs on but two subjects—his belief that he is fully sane and should be released, and his obsession that he is the victim of machinations on the part of everyone.

I know this so I have avoided him. He is confined in one of the wards devoted to those for whom there is no chance for recovery. But a few patients from that ward are permitted to go to the park, just as are some of us on the "best" ward. It was at the park that Simonds managed to corner me.

He drew me aside, urgently. "I want to talk to you about something very important, both to yourself and to me," he said. "It is particularly about myself. You know, of course, that I was brought here through a damnable conspiracy. I can prove this the moment I am brought before any board or body of men which is not controlled by my former wife's family, or my other enemies. Just put me through any tests. See if I am not fully sane."

He caught my arm in a convulsive grip. "They have followed me here. They have posted men on my ward, masquerading as patients. But I have them spotted. I know them. See that man there? He is here only to watch me."

I changed the subject at every conceivable opportunity. But it had no effect; he was right back on it in a moment.

I asked him why he does not write while he is confined here. "Why of course I couldn't do that," he replied. "I have to watch. I don't have time to write. I have to watch every minute."

I let him talk to me for half an hour. Just before the attendant called to him to fall into line and march back to his ward he placed his lips close to my ear and whispered: "Let me warn you; you can't trust anybody. Watch every man and woman. They might not be after you, but they might try to hurt you because you have been friendly to me."

Poor Old Man Simonds! He is about sixty years old. He has failed rapidly since he has been here. It won't be long now.

Some forms of insanity become more pronounced as time passes. There is Louis the Talker. Louis is not on the receiving ward with the "better patients" now. He has forfeited the privilege. He developed quarrelsome traits. He clashed with other patients and defied attendants. For a time they overlooked this, but after he had had several fights with patients and two or three with attendants he was sent to a ward for more violent inmates. There he is kept locked in his room. He is not permitted to go to the dining room for his meals; he is too provocative. His meals are taken to him.

"That's the way," snarls Hilton, the argumentative, insulting epileptic; the fellow whom nobody likes. "They put a crazy man here to make him get crazier. That's just the way they go."

Hilton, himself, is nominally confined to his room, now. But the attendants on this ward are too kind hearted to keep him locked up during this hot weather. They keep his door unlocked and open, but make him stay within the confines of his room unless he is going to the bathroom or wash room. His meals are brought to him.

We, the other patients, would like to see Hilton transferred. He will hurl unprovoked insults at patients who happen to pass by his open door. His very infrequent attempts to be pleasant are changed into irritating snarls by his mental quirk. But the hospital authorities keep him on this ward. There's a reason.

"We don't dare put him on any other ward," one of the officials said. "The patients on any ward but this one would kill him." We admit that—but we could see Hilton started for the roughest ward in the hospital without shedding a tear or harboring even the teeniest regret. Shame on me!

I just heard about the woman who tried to commit suicide and failed. "She twisted her bed sheet, tied one end to the bars at the top of the window in her room, climbed up on the window, tied the other end around her neck and jumped off," an attendant told me. "But she had left so much slack that her feet reached the floor before the sheet tightened around her throat.

"They got her before she could try it again. Since she made a bad job of it I don't believe any of the other suicidals will try it, but if she had made a go of it half the suicidals on the ward would have tried the same thing before morning.

"It's funny about these suicidals. Just let one of them manage to kill himself someway and the others who hear of it will try the same thing if you don't watch them. And the news spreads to other wards and pretty soon you have a regular epidemic of suicide tries." Other attendants tell me this is true.

The screams from the ward below this and from the Hydro come mostly from several patients recently received. Until the last two weeks we have had no "squallers" among incoming patients for a long time. But two of those just arrived make up for the slack interim.

One is an old man, very bony and with a tight drawn, parchment-like skin. There is something the matter with his spine, so that he can not use his legs. He is compelled to lie in bed. His voice is high pitched and piercing. If anyone so much as opens the door of his room the old man starts screaming. "Don't hurt me! Don't hurt me! Oh-oooO! Don't kill me. Oh-oooO!"

His terrified shrieks would lead any listener to believe that he is being torn limb from limb, but his outbreak may be caused by someone bringing him a meal, or even by a patient glancing in through the little square opening in the door of his room.

His terror seems to give him a false courage after he has finally decided that whoever has entered his room is not going to hurt him. Then he will swear horribly and make alarming threats. Some of the patients seem to enjoy gazing through the door opening and listening to him, when the attendants are not near. The old man is helpless on his bed, and knows it. But he will screamingly beg for his "Winchester." "I'll kill everybody in this—place if I can get my Winchester," he will rave. "What kind of a blankety-blank-blank place is this, anyhow? Oo-oooO! Don't hurt me! Don't hurt me! You blankety-blank-blanks. Just come in reach of my two hands. I can tear any two of you to pieces if I just get my hands on you. Oh-oooO! Don't kill me."

The other squaller is being treated in the Hydro, two floors below this. We have never seen him, but how we have heard him. He has a voice which would make an Ozark hog-caller turn green with envy. He gives tongue to but two different cries, preferring to stick closely to those he has practiced and in which he excels.

Either one of them, given with his customary earnestness, would scare all the racketeers out of Chicago. "Eee-EEE-Yow-EEE-eee!" His voice begins with the first wail of a steam siren, increases in volume, breaks into a great explosion of sound, then gradually dies away as if the siren were losing its force. His other call begins with a "Wa-hoo-eee" which rocks the building, and winds up with an "Ah-YOW-Eee" which drops bumpety-bumping down the stairs and ends in the basement. Nights, between the call of "bed time" and the hour when we get up, are his favorite practice periods.

When my neuritis is not keeping me painfully awake I have learned, at last, to sleep through ordinary outbreaks. Some of the older patients seem never to hear them. But when these two recruits join in with the nightly feminine chorus sleep flees in panic from my room.

The terrified "Don't hurt me. Don't kill me!" of the older man is the worst. His terror sounds so real.

"A fear complex. He can't help it," one of the physicians says. The attendants have a different opinion. "Just pure cussedness," is their verdict. I am told that his wife took care of him for two years after he began raving in this way, refusing to let friends have him committed to the asylum. I hereby award her a distinguished service cross and a medal for self-sacrificing heroism.

One of the several patients who are having disturbed spells is the state checker champion; which means no disrespect to other checker players. It could be no dishonor to be beaten by a player of his uncanny ability. A score of other patients here are excellent checker players. They have so little else to do that they play by the hour every day. Two or three of them have carefully cherished books of checker problems, which they study religiously. The average player would have little chance with them, but in turn they have no chance with the champion. He sits down to a game, with a bored look, and in a few apparently unconsidered moves usually clear the board of his opponent's men. Yet he is incurably insane.

Ordinarily he is trusted with several duties. He brings the meals to those on the ward who are not permitted to go to the dining room. He is in charge of keeping the stairways spotlessly clean. He is a willing worker. Now he flocks by himself; mouthing unintelligible mutterings. He will talk to no one unless it is to "mooch" tobacco, cigarette papers, candy or fruit. Even then his eyes are smoldering—suspicious of every one.

He is the most inveterate and incurable moocher on the ward. He became such a continual pest in begging me for tobacco that a harum-scarum young patient and myself set an unkind trap for him. We took a partly filled can of tobacco and dosed it liberally with red pepper, set it in plain view on the bureau in my room, then went out and waited to see what would happen.

In order to know when the trap had been sprung we set the can on some scraps of paper and opened the window so that the breeze could blow in. When we came back to the room we found the scraps of paper scattered about the room and the can of peppered tobacco sitting in a different place from where we had set it. Some one had taken the bait.

We found the checker champion sitting on the exercising porch. His pipe was still hot but he was not smoking it. Sweat was pouring off his face and he was drawing big breaths of cold air into his mouth in gulps. We did not have the heart to tease him. But my tobacco has been safe ever since; the news spread to all the moochers on the ward.

Now that he has a disturbed spell I am apprehensively wondering if he remembers that peppered tobacco. I am not frightened; certainly not. But I manage to sidle toward my room if I catch him glaring at me.

My room, though, is no sanctuary from my thoughts, my grim introspections, my unsolved problems. Like grinning gibbons they cling to the walls of my room and jeer me.

"Which way out?" they jibe. I have no answer.

Hard Common Sense stalks stolidly in and seats himself in my other chair. (I have managed to get an extra one.) A stooped, haggard fellow, who bears some resemblance to the Better Self I used to claim, drags in and seats himself on my bed. The three of us engage in a three sided argument which is never settled.

"You can not introduce her to your mother, your sister, your brothers or your friends. She is just not your kind." Common Sense opens his barrage.

"She pulled you back from the brink. She writes to you, visits you, thinks of ways to make you happier," retorts Better Self.

"You can not make her happy; you would only make both of you miserable; only insure you both of a bitter hell," Common Sense shouts.

Better Self points an accusatory finger. "That is not Common Sense talking to you. That is Cowardice, in a cheating masquerade."

There is a stir in the hall. "Packages," shouts an attendant. One of them is for me; from her. Cakes and candies. My tormentors have not moved in their seats. Better Self is watching me narrowly. Common Sense charges back to the attack.

"You have to whip Booze and the world when you go home. With her you can't whip either of them."

I thrust the package away from me. "I have not whipped Booze yet," I tell them, despondently.

"Party woman. Just a party woman. A hotel woman. Just that and nothing more." Common Sense snorts. "You are both too old to change. She could never be your kind. You could never be hers."

Better Self speaks softly. "Ask yourself what you owe her."

"Owe her?" Common Sense snaps back. "When from the first you have forbidden her to write to you or see you?. When everything she has done for you has been due to a woman's determination to get what she wants? Would you better either her or yourself?"

I raise my head and start to speak.

Out in the hall the attendant switches on the lights although it is not quite dusk. "Bed time," he shouts imperatively. My companions have vanished. The light routed them. The jibing gibbons have gone. I prepare for bed.

I slump down on the sheets. Outside rises the nightly chorus of shrieks, curses, wild screams. Piercing it all rises the cry of the old man with the fear complex. "Don't hurt me! Don't hurt me! Oh-OOO! Don't kill me!" Whizbang Mabel swings in with her mighty bellowing of new and unused obscenities. My head is hot.

Suddenly the shouting and the tumult dies. There comes one of those inexplicable pauses when the forces of bedlam draw breath and gird themselves for greater efforts. Through the momentary quiet a woman's voice rises in an old hymn. I know it. Every word of its opening lines cuts through the jumbling chaos in my mind and pricks itself into my consciousness:

"Which way shall I take? Shouts a voice on the night.
I'm a pilgrim aweary, and spent is my light."

The tumult crashes out again; blots out the voice of the singer.
Which way shall I take?

CHAPTER XIV

The Sterilization Spectre

THE patients on the receiving ward are in seething unrest. The two thousand men and women in the institution are in a foment. I suspect that this is true in every asylum in the state, and to a minor degree in the state school for the feeble-minded, although many of the boys and girls in that institution are not old enough to appreciate the situation.

The spectre of sex sterilization has been thrust over us. The legislature has passed and the governor has signed a measure permitting the desexualization, under certain conditions, of any male or female inmate who is not too aged to procreate.

And the patients are frightened, wrought up, angry and muttering. They know little about the law, therefore they are the more frightened. Men and women fear most that of which they know the least. And the patients know only what the newspapers have told them.

Into every ward of the hospital some daily papers come. Many of the patients are regular subscribers to papers from their home city and religiously read every item in every issue. But the subject of sex sterilization is avoided like a plague by most newspapers. Their editors are afraid of offending some narrow or prudish reader, so such vital facts are largely avoided.

Knowing so little the patients are the more frightened and angry, expecting the worst. They gather in little knots and discuss the fate which may be hanging over them. But they do not do it where the attendants can hear. They are afraid to do that.

"The paper says they can sterilize any male patient under sixty-five years old and any female under forty-seven. That seems nearly all of us, even to the little children," one patient says in helpless anger. "If they do that to me they might as well kill me and be done with it. If they don't I'll kill myself anyhow. I haven't got much to live for as it is but if they do that I won't give a damn what becomes of me." I really think this man means it. I know that he believes he means it.

"Well if they do that to me I'll kill the man who orders it done if it takes me the rest of my life." The patient who says this has always been a quiet man, obedient and likable. It is difficult to determine that he is insane. Yet I am told that he comes exactly in one of the classifications intended to be reached by the sterilization law. He is abnormally sexed. "Well I know what I'm agoing to do. I'm not agoing to stay here," another patient says. His sentiments are echoed fervently by numerous others. And that is just one of the reasons why the sterilization law, as passed, will defeat its own purpose. It will lead—is already leading—to desperate attempts at escape. Some of these will be successful.

The fear of the law has already led to one successful effort to escape, on this ward alone. A parole man, sub-witted but considered harmless, became so worried that he made a successful break for freedom. He is still at large, capable of fathering children and with that thought indubitably brought uppermost in his mind. "I am going right back to my country girl," he has since written to one of the other patients here. Had he not been frightened by the passage of the law very probably he would still be here where there is no possibility of his even associating with the other sex.

There is another way, far, far more serious, in which the law will defeat its purpose. Many families have members who are idiotic, epileptic, feeble-minded, imbecile or even possessed of mental quirks, and under former circumstances they would not have hesitated to have these unfortunates confined; but now they will avoid having them committed, no matter what the cost in deception, risk

Thus many persons who should be confined will be at large with the possibility of bringing about reproduction. And many of them will be of two types that the measure is especially designed to reach—either suffering from the effects of social diseases, or abnormally sexed. In both of these classes it is extremely difficult for the layman to determine when the point of insanity is reached, so that if the victim does not in some way come under the observation of competent physicians he may remain at large for long periods without his casual associates realizing that he is abnormal. There lies the danger to society.

Personally I am not so seriously concerned about the law. I have studied it and know its provisions. I obtained from the ward physician special permission to obtain a copy, but the permission was granted on the strict condition that I would not discuss it with the other patients or even let them know that I have it. I would not do the latter even if permitted to do so, as the other patients would almost mob me to get an opportunity to read it. Then many of them would not be able to understand it and the frightened discussions would start all over again.

Those patients most deeply steeped in delusions are the worst excited. "The paper says that the superintendent decides whether you are to be sterilized or not. Of course he will pick on me right away. He's always had a grudge against me. He's only keeping me here for spite, anyway," one of them says.

He is right in one thing. The law does leave the decision as to whether or not a patient is to be sterilized to the superintendent, practically alone, although it was not intended to do exactly that. It errs most in its assumption that the men who administer it will be trained, conscientious, and, above all else, infallibly capable in judgment. But are laws always administered by such super-perfect humans? I am leaving out of all consideration the question of whether society ever has the right to inflict sterilization.

I am leaving that question to the churches and the consciences of the people. Some of the greatest of the churches have taken an unyielding stand against any sterilization. I am not discussing whether it would be right to inflict sterilization for something of which the helpless victim is not willfully guilty. And I admit that at first reading and on first thought the law might appear to be a good one for society at large; but a closer analysis shows it to be as full of holes as a fish net; presenting uncounted opportunities for tragic travesties on right while giving the perpetrators the protection of being within the law.

The first section of the law provides that the superintendents of asylums "when they are of the opinion that it is for the best interests of society and of the patients, may perform or cause to be performed the operation of sterilization on any such patients afflicted with hereditary forms of insanity, which are recurrent—idiocy, imbecility, feeble-mindedness or epilepsy."

This section contains the gist of the law; remaining sections being devoted to an outline of legal and medical steps required, including legal steps by which the patient, supposedly, may protect himself.

The measure has been intentionally provided with several "legal safeguards,"—but these are such that they can be of use only to those who are *mentally* and *financially* capable of taking advantage of them.

These steps include a hearing before the board of control and a possible appeal to the state courts. The patient must bear all the expense and burden of his appeals; the superintendent's "opinion" is supported by the state's attorney general, and the state treasury defrays any court or other expense which the superintendent may incur.

"That's no protection at all to any of us," Borden says bitterly. Borden was an excellent architect while outside. "We are either actual or legal paupers and can't hire attorneys, and we are either insane and can't look out for ourselves, or everybody who might help us believes we are insane because we are here, which has the same effect."

"You're right," says Whitney, a former farmer. "Then we are completely shut in. We can't even send out a letter if they don't want us to." (This is true. Officials have turned down several letters which I have written to outside friends, and I can not guess or discover the reason.)

"We can not use a telephone," Whitney continues. "We can not send out a telegram without special permission, and they never give us that. We are hedged in; practically buried. Then we are flat broke. I have money and property at home but I can't use either one. My wife is my administrator and she is running around with another fellow, and she and my grown son both want my farm. What could I do if they wanted to sterilize me?"

Because I have read the law I can tell him what he can do. He can stay here until he dies, whether he recovers or not, whether he is sane or insane, if the superintendent should decide that he should be sterilized. Unless he submitted to the mutilation that decision of the doctor's would rob him of all hope of ever going home. Even the reformers who forced the passage of the law realized that there is no possibility of offspring as long as the patient is shut up here; so the measure provides that only patients "about to be discharged" may be forced to submit to sterilization.

Does that mean that a man may be sane enough to be discharged and yet insane enough to be forced to submit to sterilization against his will?

"How are they going to know what forms of insanity can be passed on to the children?" Borden asks. "Even the doctors in this hospital don't agree on that. They are going to let the superintendent's opinion force men to be sterilized, and all superintendents don't agree on what can be transmitted. That law is rotten, but it has been passed and what can we do about it. None of us can go into court and fight it. Most of us haven't a dime and those of us who have estates can't use them. Our administrators wouldn't let us."

Borden is correct in both of his conclusions. The best informed physicians are sharply divided in opinion as to what forms of insanity are transmittable; and administrators, as a rule, will not advance funds for a long and expensive court fight to save the patient from sterilization. They will take the position that "The doctor surely must know what is best."

There is a patient on this ward who owns an estate said to be valued at about $1,000,000. If he were about to be released and the superintendent should decide that he should first be sterilized would his administrator or his prospective heirs advance money to fight the matter through the courts and thus set him at liberty? Or would they not rather insist that he should not be released without sterilization. They would know that he would resist sterilization and thus be forced to remain in the asylum.

It would tear up their pretty playhouse so rudely if he should be discharged and permitted to resume control of his affairs; especially after the prospective heirs have it all arranged among them just how the big estate is to be divided, and the administrator has decided that his nice, fat job is good for several years.

Such injustices are particularly apt to occur when the husband or wife has been instrumental in having the patient committed. In many such cases the husband or wife does not want the patient discharged.

A lover, sweetheart, the estate or even physical fear may be the reason. But no matter what the reason, the outside spouse seldom will be willing to supply the money to carry on the expensive court fight which would be required to overthrow the superintendent's decision. As for the patients themselves, they have no money except what little is sent to some of them, and even this must be spent under supervision. I have a little money in a bank at home but I can not draw a cent of it, even "tobacco money."

The framers of the law evidently believed it was "fully safeguarded." I am convinced that the men who passed the laws permitting the execution of death sentences on witches and those under which heretics were burned at the stake believed that those laws were "fully safeguarded."

Later knowledge has proved how completely illogical those safeguards were, but that does not return life to the innocent victims. And the person of today who advocates the sterilization of men and women, boys and girls—when no physician can say with certainty what insanities can be transmitted to offspring, may be putting himself in the same class with the burners of witches.

Today the famous Salem witchcraft obsession is referred to by some physicians as a "mass mania or insanity." Their predecessors were no doubt called into court to testify as to whether or not the accused persons were possessed of "witches' minds."

Certain it is that records, still existing, show that among the witnesses in several cases were a "leech and a minister." And now I know from what sources some of the criminal court alienists of today were derived.

The informed medical profession of today is sharply divided on the question of what forms of insanity are the result of heredity. Formerly practically all physicians were agreed that the vast majority of insanity cases were the result of heredity. Even within the last year I have had a bombastic general physician tell me that "ninety per cent of insanity can be traced to heredity."

Of course this man was ridiculously wrong. He knew nothing of insanity or insane persons. He had no business talking on the subject. But many people who hear him make such ridiculous statements will believe him, because, "Doctor Pomposity said so; I heard him myself." And a few hundred years ago all of the Doctor Pompositys said—and so the people believed—that insane persons were possessed of an evil spirit. So the victims were chained up and starved to drive out the evil spirits. Those must have been stubborn spirits; they always refused to leave until after their hosts died.

But even those physicians who make a scientific study of insanity, and are in no way kin to Doctor Pomposity, are divided into two classes on the subject of the transmissibility of insanity. One class, which is growing smaller, holds that the majority of insanity cases can be traced to heredity. The other class holds that in many cases formerly ascribed to heredity the transmission certainly can not be proved, and is very doubtful; while the majority of insanity cases may be due to organic physical ailments, social or other germ diseases, injuries, and a variety of other causes, including nervous shock or tension; as witness the religious maniacs, victims of so-called shell shock or of worry, and women who become demented from the nervous and physical strains of childbirth.

With the best informed doctors failing to agree can the conscientious person contend that the mere opinion of a physician should be permitted to determine if a lifelong mutilation should be imposed on other persons? If so, to which class of physicians should we listen? And is it certain that the superintendent who must pass on the cases will happen to belong to that class? Even physicians in the same hospital often are divided. They are very much so here.

Regardless of the hazy ideas of such laymen as happen to know what the terms mean, and equally regardless of a very few physicians who are almost as uninformed, vasectomy in the case of males and salpingectomy in the case of females is mutilation; uninformed statements to the contrary notwithstanding. Original claims for these two forms of sterilization, which are the only two permitted under the law, were that sexual association is not eliminated but that procreation is. But calm statistics show that a very high percentage of the operations fail to attain this result and surgeons are beginning to admit that very much of the attraction of a woman for a man or of a man for a woman is irretrievably lost even in the most successful operations. And this attraction is the basis of affection between the sexes which keeps households together and families happy.

The divorce laws of practically every state recognize this when they make sterility of one of the contracting parties a good and sufficient ground for divorce.

As for the provision in the law that the patient must be notified in advance and a hearing held by the board of control before the sterilization can be carried out, that is of little if any protection. The patient can not represent himself successfully; he requires an attorney, alienists and perhaps other witnesses.

The members of the board usually are politicians or business men; they know nothing of insanity, and have had no opportunity to study the patient; they haven't an idea as to what forms of insanity are transmittable.

They will naturally and almost unvaryingly rely on the word of the superintendent; the very same superintendent who has already decided that the patient should be sterilized and who will be present to uphold his opinion.

If the members of the board attempted to cross-examine the patient they would be prone to some ludicrous mistakes. Many badly insane persons are apparently sane, rational and keen when they are not having one of their disturbed periods. At such times they would deceive the very elect, while a harmless person with the mentality of a child would be trapped by the veriest tyro. The board members, knowing this, would rely on the recommendation of the superintendent, and the superintendent could overbalance any good impression that the patient had made by simply tapping his head or winking significantly.

After the hearing before the board the patient, although pronounced by the superintendent as sane and ready to go out into the world, would have to remain in the asylum unless he submits to sterilization or appeals to the courts. In not one per cent of the cases would the patient be able to appeal to the courts. He could not obtain the necessary money. He could not communicate with friends if the superintendent did not wish him to do so. Even if he communicates with them they are not apt to come to his aid, in the face of the decision of the superintendent and the board. They would believe the authorities were right. Certainly they would not advance large sums out of their own pocket. Would you, even if it were your brother who had been pronounced insane?

Depending on the opinion of a physician is natural. The most hard headed, and sanest, people do it to a surprising degree. Men frequently give up their positions or sell their businesses and move to a different climate on the advice of their physician. And in mental cases the unquestioning dependence of people on the word of a physician is almost absolute.

Of course the framers of the law contend that the superintendents of the hospitals, who are very often political appointees, will be conscientious in giving their opinion that patients should be sterilized. Unquestionably many of them will. The "leech and minister" were undoubtedly conscientious in giving their opinions that the poor Salem wretches had witches' minds. And even where the superintendent is scrupulously conscientious in giving his opinion the fact remains that it is but an opinion and later knowledge may prove it to have been unjustified.

And the assumption of the proponents of the law that such opinions will be honestly given in all cases can not be justified by part experience. The human element creeps through all such assumptions of law. Are not judgeships sometimes bought? Are all verdicts uninfluenced? Do all contracts go to the lowest and best bidder? Is the Volstead law always conscientiously enforced? Are not the gods of money, politics and selfishness some times served?

Is there not a possibility that some superintendent might be influenced by surgeons coveting the fee which the state will pay to the surgeons performing the operations?

No better refutation of the claim that superintendents will never apply the law except where abundantly justified need be offered than the proved fact that, in the past, superintendents of some hospitals, without a scintilla of law to justify them, secretly have sterilized helpless and hapless patients. They used the barbarous method of removing some of the reproductive organs, just as is done with colts or calves. Not only was there no law to permit this; the action was directly against the law. But the superintendents evidently depended upon the fact that their word is law within their domains, and patients are helpless.

More than twenty-five years ago there was an infamous case of this in Kansas where the superintendent of one of the state hospitals sterilized not merely one but a considerable number of patients and endeavored to keep the matter secret. But some of the patients managed to get out of the hospital and their mutilation was proof of their stories. The brutal superintendent is said to have justified his action on the ground that it was in the interest of scientific knowledge, and that the men and women whom he mutilated were "just crazy people, anyhow."

He was discharged from his position, but did that right the great wrong which he had committed? It has been charged that physicians and superintendents in many hospitals for the insane have used patients, or permitted them to be used, for experimental operations of different kinds. In some instances these charges have been authenticated.

One of the physicians here, with whom I have discussed the law at length, admits the measure has many faults, but is a staunch advocate of a law permitting sterilization in certain cases, provided it is thoroughly safeguarded. Most of the other physicians are in accord with him, and I believe they are conscientious and sincere.

I might agree with them—if such a law could be properly safeguarded. But I believe this is impossible under present lack of definite knowledge concerning insanity, and is almost impossible so long as superintendents of hospitals are subject to political appointment.

In this institution there formerly was a physician of such odor that I hold my nose when I think of him. He did not last very long. He was abruptly discharged—and kicked up a political row about it.

Yet during the time he was here he stood in the capacity of a hospital physician, and relatives of patients accepted his word unquestioningly. He was culpably incompetent, fundamentally dishonest and constitutionally unconscientious. Yet he could have caused untold injustice by a few words or by merely tapping his head.

But the physician who believes in legal sterilization in certain rare cases has given considerable thought to the subject and has evolved a plan which many good people will endorse.

He would permit no sterilization without a hearing before a board composed in part of legally trained men, in part of laymen, preferably substantial business men, and in part of physicians who are experienced in mental cases but are not connected with the institution in which the patient is confined. The state commissioner of charities and corrections would be, ex officio, defender of the patient, empowered to call witnesses and alienists at state expense. Such a board might possibly be able to reach a just conclusion and the patient automatically would have some one charged with and empowered to represent his interests.

"There are," says this physician, "Some women, excellent wives and mothers, who, due to the nervous and physical strains of childbirth, become mentally deranged. After they are here for a time they recover, mentally and physically. But their next childbirth results in a recurrence of the mental derangement.

"Would it not be better if they should be sterilized and so be able to go home, take care of their children and be useful homemakers than for them to be permitted to bear more children at the expense of dementia on their part, leaving the children uncared for and essentially motherless?"

Right, in some ways, Doctor. But if she again is sane as you claim, if she is mentally competent to go home to her husband and children and be a good homemaker and credit to her family, is she not competent to pass on the question of her own sterilization? Should not that question be left to herself, her husband and her conscience?

And should it not be decided where the threat of having to remain in the asylum, coupled with her yearning for her children, home, husband and freedom, can not beat her down into despairing acceptance?

But the doctor is not through with the presentation of his case. "There are some men in the asylums who are children in mentality, but physically they are adults, capable of procreating children. Their families are able and willing to care for them and support them. Also it is cruel to keep them confined here in association with those who are irrevocably deranged. Would not it be better that they should be sterilized and sent home than that they should be kept virtual prisoners for something for which they are not responsible?"

Right again, in some ways, Doctor. But if your theory that idiocy is always transmittable is correct, should not the other members of his family, his brothers and sisters be sterilized also? They unquestionably must have inherited some of the taint from the same source from which he received his. They come from the same father and mother, the same ancestry. And shall we sterilize his father and mother? They have produced one idiot child, hence may produce another. The idiot, at least has not done this and there is no proof that he may.

If the theory of transmitted idiocy is correct the parents' tendency to produce idiotic children has been proved. Shall we let them go and sterilize the child they brought into the world?

Shall we say that when an idiot makes his appearance in a family all members of that family should be sterilized? Inherited traits sometimes skip a generation. Shall we sterilize his grandfather? And what about cousins, second, third and umpty-fourth cousins? Where does the taint end?

And can those unanalytical reformers who shout vigorously and vociferously for sterilization and who stampede legislatures, be assured that some twenty-second cousin of their own was not born feeble-minded?

Such a logical interpretation of your theory of hereditary idiocy would be apt to cause an awful furor among our best people, would it not, Doctor? Some of the most prominent families in the country have produced feebleminded children. They hide them away with the other family skeletons. And have not many families of apparently low intelligence produced some mental giants? Whence came Lincoln?

How about new blood to bolster up our civilization at intervals. Must it come only from those of our present mental heavyweights who can trace their ancestry back to Noah, including all the family branches and ramifications, to show that no insanity, imbecility, idiocy or feeble-mindedness ever tainted the blood?

Shall we automatically divorce couples when it can be shown that one of the parties is a member of a family which has at some time produced a child which was not up to mental par? And what constitutes mental par?

There are men who are idiotic or insane from injuries, pre-natal or since birth. How can the physician know? Shall we sterilize them?

But while I have been getting myself all hot and bothered about the matter the other patients on the ward are more than hot and bothered. They are frightened and dreading.

They congregate on the exercising porch and talk about it. Through mysterious grapevine sources we have learned that the women are as wrought up as the men. Perhaps they are more so. Strip from any woman all her overgarments of training, repression, pretension and artifice and you will find that her thoughts are of the other sex. Her dreams and her life are expressed in terms of the masculine gender. Sweetheart, husband, lover or perhaps a son; her real life is wrapped up in these. A man has other interests; he can immerse himself in business or hobbies. He is, often, quite willing to live alone in a club, hotel or even a boarding house. A woman is not, even in this age of flappers and business women.

The modern flapper has thrust aside repressions and is striving for "self expression," which usually includes calling up a boy friend and inviting him on a necking party. If he is "dated up" or not interested she has little hesitancy in calling another one. And all of us here know where the minds of older women swing when their restraints are loosened or erased by mental unbalance. Yes, the women are worried about the sterilization law.

Those here think, talk and dream about little else but men. They crowd to their barred windows and flirt shamelessly with anything in trousers which happens to pass near their wards. Their advances are bold, bald and urging.

And so the fears, the loneliness and the near-hopelessness of the locked-ins have an added terror.

Its poignancy will wear off to some extent as time goes on and the patients learn of no sterilizations; for they will never learn of any which are performed, unless it be through some mischance. Nor will the public.

But, knowing my insane associates, I know that each new patient who may be brought in will be warned of the possible fate which awaits him, and his hopes will be even fewer than were those of us older patients who heard the click of the lock in the heavy door before the sterilization law was passed.

CHAPTER XV

IN SELF DEFENSE

RUDD, who has had a grounds parole for two months, was brought back on the receiving ward yesterday. This morning they took him to Ward J. That means he will be kept locked up in a tight little sideroom as long as he is there.

For Rudd has gone blooie. To make it plainer, he has turned bughouse. To make it still plainer, he has cracked.

They often do that, under the effects of the life here, even when they come in perfectly sane.

Rudd is the fellow who had the expensive family and who conspired to have himself committed in order to escape conviction for selling mortgaged property, after the stock-market debacle wiped out his house of cards. The man he had defrauded had influence. He knew that Rudd was not insane and through devious ways he managed to have him returned to his home county for trial on a criminal charge.

But the members of the jury which tried him were just like the rest of the men and women outside. Rudd had been declared insane by physicians, therefore they believed him insane. He was sent back here.

The hospital authorities at once put him on parole. They knew he was not insane.

Why, he was as sane as I am. —— Is that a snicker I hear?

So Rudd went to work in the hospital store. His business training and experience were valuable there. He became almost indispensable to the store keeper and the hospital steward.

But during his stay outside while he was awaiting trial he had suffered a tremendous shock to his self esteem.

When first he was committed here he was a prominent business man of the little city in which he lived. He had built whole flocks of residences and sold them on the monthly payment plan. He had been president of a civic club and active in the chamber of commerce. His wife belonged to several exclusive women's organizations, and lovingly and assiduously polished her social standing every day, to keep it bright. His son and daughter were attending exclusive schools. When the business crash swept away the pyramided credits of his building operations his frantic efforts to enable his family to keep up with the Smythes and the Brownes led him to sell some of his holdings without first paying off the encumbrances.

He had done this before when credits were easy. Of course it was technically wrong—but then he was a prominent citizen, a town builder, and certainly no one would charge such a man as himself with crime over a little detail of business. And as long as he strained his credit and paid off the indebtedness later it was perfectly all right. Certainly, also, the financing concerns wanted to keep their money busy, the money which hard working people had entrusted to them for safe investment,—and Rudd was keeping it busy for them.

But Rudd learned something. What is only technically wrong in times of elastic credits may be very, very wrong when credits contract. The financing concerns took fright at the credit collapse. It was all right for Rudd to be so careless previously, and they had purred when he later paid off the mortgages. But now one man filed stern charges. So Rudd's attorney advised him to be committed here.

But when Rudd went back for trial he learned something else. His wife decidedly was not happy to see him. His daughter and son openly avoided him; shunned him. You see he could not support them in the way to which they had been accustomed.

He had fallen down on the one job to which they always had mentally assigned him. Then, too, he had let himself be declared insane. Why, by doing that he had hurt their social standing terribly.

No, they did not rally round in his hour of need. Quite the contrary. His wife virtuously told the reporters that she was "standing by him." That looked well in the daily papers. It let other people know how loyal and self-sacrificing she was. It was "wonderful of Virginia Rudd." All the women in her clubs said so. And they all sympathized with her when she filed suit for divorce immediately after the prosecution had collapsed and Rudd was returned here, on the ground that he was insane. Of course no woman likes to remain married to an insane man—and besides he could not support her any longer.

She will not get that divorce, law and human nature being what they are. In this state the insanity of a spouse is not sufficient grounds for divorce. She alleges that he is sane and always has been so. But the judge who hears the ease will reflect that Rudd twice has been held insane. He will preach a little homily and deny the divorce.

But the fact that she filed the suit, coupled with the attitude of his son, daughter and former friends when he went back for trial, let Rudd see where he stands in the minds of others. Now, when the screams of women and the howling of squallers keep him awake nights he must brood bitterly on the thought of his desertion by those for whom he made desperate sacrifices.

Under such circumstances phrenetic worry leads straight to psychosis. We have known that Rudd was slipping. His conversation became jerky, irritable and slightly wild. This wildness increased, but still he was able to attend to his duties, at the store. His eyes became nervously bright and he avoided every one.

So we were not surprised when suddenly he went ravingly insane, yesterday morning. Now they are taking him to Ward J. A new man is working at the store.

"That's the way they go," Lawton snorts. "Keep a sane man housed up in here with a bunch of howling nuts and it makes him go crazy. Why he wasn't crazy when they brought him here. He was just as sane as I am."

"Sure," says Manning; "He was just as sane as I am."

Manning is a genial, roly-poly, happy natured man who always has a good word for everyone. He appears to be perfectly sane and sensible in every way. For weeks after he arrived I studied him, trying to find out in what way he was irrational. Finally I stooped to asking the one question which always brings out a man's delusions, here. I asked him who had had him committed.

"It was my son," he answered. "But of course they bribed him. They were afraid of my invention."

That started him, and he told me about his "invention." "I've been working on it for years," he told me. "And I have perfected it. With my discovery of a new principle you can manufacture the equipment to heat and light a five roomed house for about $28, and can operate it at an expense for both heating and lighting the entire house of not more than $2, in five years. Of course the big utilities people and the bankers would not permit me to put it on the market. It would have ruined all their investments and bankrupted them and all their stockholders. So they got to my son in some way and bribed him to have me sent here.

"They may be able to keep me here all my life, damn them. But they will never get my secret. It'll die with me. They can't get it out of me."

Now I know why Manning is here. On any other subject he is—just as sane as I am.

Then there is Stewart. He is not the least insane, and in business shrewdness he outclasses all the rest of us, even if we do not endorse his principles—or lack of them. He is so shrewd that he is actually accumulating an increasing financial nest egg while locked up on the receiving ward of a state hospital. That is being crazy like a fox.

Plodding business men will be shouldered aside when young Stewart receives his final parole. And be will get it within a few months. He is not at all the type to "go blooie" through a little thing like being confined in an insane asylum. The world, inside or out, is his oyster, and he intends to eat his oyster, seasoned just to his taste.

He is a shining product of the don't-give-a-hang jazz age, which now shows some signs of disappearing. His father is a prominent physician in a large city. He was much too busy becoming prominent to give his son any attention during his formative boyhood years. And his wife was too busy keeping her name in the Sunday society notes, and taking care of her discreet flirtations at the same time, to think about the boy.

So he just scrambled into youth; handsome, reckless, shrewd and totally inconsiderate of others. He never completed his high school course; he was too busy dizzily whizzing some flapper or young divorcee around in a big sedan, being the life of wild parties, sowing uncounted wild oats, and breaking the Mann act in half a dozen states. How the girls and women loved his daring recklessness. They were captivated by this jazz-age youngster who "knew as much as a man of thirty" yet was so irrepressibly young.

His father raged and stormed, but paid the unauthorized checks which the boy drew on his bank account, bailed him out after bad scrapes—and let him off with a lecture. Finally he abruptly balked at paying any more forged checks. Stewart gaily ran away to new scenes. California beckoned, and he never could resist any beckoning hand.

He spent four wildly reckless years out there. Lack of money never could decrease his ebullience. When nothing else was to be done he always could get a job in a restaurant, soda fountain, and pressing shop or filling station, and he could beat board and lodging bills with blithe unconcern. And on the occasions when his letters managed to wheedle his father into temporarily relenting and sending him a check he could, and did, cut a flash for a time until the money was gone—more than gone.

Then with a gay, "Oh well; what the hell?" he just went out and commandeered a new job. It was an adamant employer who could refuse Stewart a job when Stewart had made up his mind to get one.

He was a natural athlete and willing to try anything, so he tried prize fighting. But since he would not train or keep himself in condition he never got beyond the preliminaries. He managed to get a job with the football team of a Pacific coast college which did not scrutinize the antecedents of its players too closely, but too many cocktail parties promptly led to his undoing there. And the time finally came when he had to leave Los Angeles. He went home. His father received him coldly and ordered him to find a job and support himself. His mother was embarked on a new and exciting flirtation and could not bother with him. So he went out and hunted up some of his former cronies and got on such an extended spree that he landed in a hospital.

Then the fact came out that during the course of his innumerable philanderings he had contracted a social disease and the spirochete had reached his spinal canal. For the first time in his life Stewart was frightened.

He appealed to his father, but the father retorted that he had brought his misfortune on himself, had flouted all advice, and would have to find his own way out of the mess. An angry and violent scene followed; so violent that Stewart threatened his father's life. His father well knew his son's reckless nature and realized that he was in danger. He filed charges of insanity and Stewart was committed here, the lunacy board taking the position that his father was a prominent physician and certainly qualified to know whether his son was insane.

With the reckless philosophy of his nature, Stewart was not downcast about the matter. Good times and bad times, money to throw at the silk-pajamaed girls, and jerking soda for a living, were all in the game of life. Besides, he pondered, in the asylum he could get free treatment of his disease and still thumb his nose at his father. He could show the "Old Man" that he could get along without anybody's grudging aid.

He scarcely had become accustomed to the ward before his shrewd mind was evolving ways and means for earning a little spending money. He did not have a cent, not even tobacco money, and his frantic quarrel with his father made it impossible to hope for help from that source. But a little money circulates among the more fortunate patients of a hospital and the attendants and physicians get salaries. All that was necessary for Stewart to do was to find a way to turn a fair amount of this money toward himself.

The patients who get small remittances from home and who wear their own clothes require laundry work, mending, and occasionally a little cleaning and pressing of suits. Attendants must have a tidy amount of such work done. With the aplomb which had always enabled him to get a job whenever he wanted one, Stewart set about corralling the valeting business of the ward.

At first he did all the work himself, including soliciting business from the officials. He was good at soliciting business. Before long he had persuaded the physicians to let him use a vacant room and he installed an electric iron, ironing board, wash tub and board, needles, thread and other necessities. Within a few weeks he had a monopoly on all the cleaning, pressing, mending, and laundry work of the patients on the ward and for many of the attendants throughout the whole institution. His prices were about half those of the shops in town, he did excellent work and then he was conveniently at hand when any official wanted a rush job of cleaning and pressing. The town is more than three miles away from the hospital grounds.

Now he simply manages the "business"; other patients do all the work for him. The income is not large, but he is at little expense. The hospital furnishes his shop room, water, heat and electricity, and I suspect that it also furnishes his soap and gasoline—without the knowledge of the superintendent. Stewart is capable of doing some shrewd "managing." His labor costs him pitifully little. He is never bothered with strikes—this is one place where the workers can not make demands on the employer. He has no competition. And at the same time the state is treating his physical condition and giving him a free living.

That might be called turning ill fortune into a profit. He now has plenty of tobacco, fruits, good food, new shirts and ties when needed, and a cash surplus which is steadily growing.

By the time that his long course of treatments is completed be expects to have enough money to give him a year's technical education in bacteriological laboratory work. He has promise of employment, at the end of that time in a big laboratory owned by one of his father's friends. Then he plans to study medicine; earning his way by working in the laboratory.

He is determined to "show the Old Man a thing or two."

He plays on the hospital baseball team, has adroitly inched his way into getting more privileges than any other patient on the ward and comes and goes about this building almost as he pleases. It pays to be as gaily shrewd and self-serving as he is, inside an asylum.

Apparently he has forgotten, blithely, the two wives he managed to acquire during his merry philandering years. I suspect that he may have overlooked the formality of getting a divorce from the first before marrying the second.

He lords it over the other patients in a recklessly high-handed way that makes the more unfortunate ones both fear and hate him. That bothers him not at all. He assumes almost as much authority over them as do the officials, and his imperiousness is not kept in check by any fear of dismissal, as is the case with attendants. The patients are sullen at his treatment of them but they do not dare resent it; he has too much influence with the attendants, and is too shrewd for ordinary patients to risk defying him. He sees to it that none of his high-handed acts are carried out while a physician is on the ward. He is quite a different fellow then. But he is piling up a resentment against himself which may break bounds some day.

He is amusedly contemptuous of this resentment. What does it matter if a set of bugs doesn't like him? They are just nuts, anyway.

At that his course of conduct may be wiser than mine. None of the other patients gather in his room to bother him; none of them harass him with their vagaries, obsessions or delusions. Their quirks do not disturb his mind in the least. He will never go insane through association with distorted minds. He is not troubled with self analysis or wearying introspections. So he is able to shake off any ingrowing self pity as a duck shakes off water.

His way may be better than mine.

He gives never a thought to the two wives he has outside, unless it is a contemptuous one. As to his lady-loves, I doubt if he can recall the names of all of them.

While, as for me, I brood constantly on the question of what is my conscientious yet wise duty toward Constance, whom, almost from the first, I have been trying to persuade, jar or even drive out of her tenacious infatuation for me. I do not love her. I do not even admire her, when I include most of her characteristics. There is so much that I can never admire. But her unswervable and self-sacrificing devotion to me has put me inescapably in her debt. That one great characteristic calls for the deepest gratitude of which I am capable.

The question which harries me is, what course of mine will be the truest gratitude and the wisest for us both?

When Stewart gets his final parole he will continue to go his recklessly inconsiderate, gay way; overriding others and trampling straight to what he wants.

Into my room daily come the quirked and the quavering, the obsession driven and the melancholia ridden. I shoo them out as gently as possible. I have not learned to be heartlessly inconsiderate of them, no matter how much I dread their presence and their confidences. They do not seem to sense my antipathy; they sense only that I do not send them scurrying.

Perhaps I need more callousness to bolster my mental self-defense mechanism. Does self preservation, the first law of nature, include defense of one's sanity as ruthlessly as the preservation of the physical body, even when it necessitates the hurting of pitiful unfortunates?

I figuratively lay down the two attitudes side by side and compare them and their results, both in here and outside.

On the outside he was a gaily rolling stone, always half way outside the law; sometimes entirely beyond its pale. He was a soda water dispenser, restaurant waiter, a conscienceless waster. He was unscrupulous with women—and popular with them. On the outside I was accounted a man of sound civic influence in spite of my excesses, one whose editorials were read and approved by thousands and whose presence on an important committee was considered to have some value.

Here, when he strides down the hallway the groups of patients divide and give him passage way. None of them trouble him with their vagaries and obsessions. They give cringing avoidance to his room.

When I go down the hallway they beg me for tobacco, for reading matter and even for money. They draw me to one side to beg me to intercede with the physicians for them so that they may go home. They corner me to tell me how unjustly they are held here when they are all right and want to go home. They make me listen to fantastic delusions.

Is right conduct a matter of environment? Do the conditions in which a man is placed decide what is the upright thing to do? Can kindly principles, which are right and wise on the outside of an asylum, become wrong and foolish on the inside?

May my better self forgive me. I am almost persuaded that the answer is—YES.

CHAPTER XVI

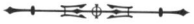

FUTILE

JOE'S mother is sick. And Joe wanders about the ward in a half-comprehending daze; or he sits in his room for hours at a time, in a sort of stunned passivity.

Joe is wondering what he will do if his mother should die, for the doctors have told him that his mother's condition, at her age, is very serious. And his mother is the only thing which Joe has; the only person or object for which he has felt any affection or even interest in all his futile, weakly stumbling fifty-two years of life.

Joe is the little man with the graying hair and weak, trembling face, whose room is just down the hall from mine. He has been here for fifteen years. But Joe does not mind. He does not mind anything, just so he is near his mother. And Joe's mother has been a patient here a little longer than he has.

Mother and son, one aged, the other past the meridian of life; both inmates in the same insane asylum, and not a known relative or friend in the great, free world outside. And Joe's mother is going to die.

Her illness and Joe's dazed stumbling about the ward have brought out a story, so strange, so somberly motivated that it arrests attention even on an insane ward. More than fifty-one years ago Joe arrived in the Indian Territory, a puny babe in his mother's arms. They came on the seat of a ranch wagon, beside Big Bill Barde, who ran thousands of cattle in the Big Pasture section of old Fort Bill, a government military post.

Big Bill had found the mother trying to earn a living of a sort for herself and child by washing dishes in an untidy restaurant in the bare little Kansas cattle town where he had gone to load his four-year-olds for shipment to the Kansas City market.

No one knew her past, where she had come from or how she had reached that out-of-the-way place. In all the after years she never told a soul, not even her son. She dated her life from the time when she appeared at the back door of that little restaurant and hesitatingly asked for something to eat. She was half starved, and the only possessions she had in the world were her child and the scanty clothing which the two of them wore. She paid for her meals by doing the dish-washing and other rough kitchen work, her baby cradled on a wooden bench, on some folded cloths.

Little Joe cried scarcely at all, and then only in a helplessly frightened way—a predication of his characteristics through life.

It was inevitable that Big Bill, who hid an almost foolishly kind heart under a rough and gruff exterior, should offer to take the two back to the ranch with him and give the mother a job as cook, although she would be the only white woman within twenty miles. It also was inevitable that she should accept, as this would give her at least some place where she could care for her child while earning a living for them both. So, seated in the wagon beside Big Bill, the two made the ten day trip to the K-Bar ranch headquarters.

The woman spoke scarcely at all during the entire trip, but she helped with the camp arrangements at night and did all the camp cooking. The baby cried little, and then only in his oddly futile way. If the mother felt any excitement, fear or other emotion she never expressed it, unless some slight change in her dull black eyes could be called expression.

Those eyes were usually brooding, with a hint of suppressed storms in them.

So began their life on the territory prairies, with only the rough but kindly cowboys for companions. The woman never noticed the men or seemed to know that they were around.

She answered never a word to their attempts at light-hearted badinage. And with the broad and understanding tolerance of the West, they soon learned that she wanted only to be let alone, and accepted her on that basis.

It was not that she ever actively rebuffed a single person; she seemed too negative for that. It was that she never felt, or seemed to feel, any interest of any kind or degree in any person or any thing except her child; and she never displayed any active emotion toward it, at least in the presence of others. She went about her work silently, ploddingly but skillfully. Storms flashed in her dull black eyes at times but she never gave way to them during those first few years.

"Must be a streak of Indian in her, somewheres, the way she holds herself in," Big Bill would muse at times. But if there were such a strain no one ever learned it. Her past remained, and still remains, sealed.

As for the boy, he grew up on that Indian Territory ranch, without playmates and with but one comrade—his mother. At the frequent attempts of the cowboys to make friends with him, to stir him to laughter or even to interest, he would stare in a half frightened way and escape to his mother as soon as possible. He almost never laughed. He showed no interest in or aptitude for any boyish sports. He never seemed to have boyish imagination or energy. Birth had made him a boy but evidently in inclination he was a frightened, silent, brooding girl, without confidences or self confidence.

"Futile!" Big Bill would snort to himself, sometimes. "Futile; that's what he is. Don't believe his mind is all there. Him and her would make a strange pair in any man's country."

So the years went on. Joe, almost unwillingly, learned to ride, to tend the horses, help with the ranch chores, even to do rough work when it was really necessary.

The men scarcely ever asked him to take a hand at haying, fence building or other work of the kind, nor did he volunteer in words. When he sensed that he was really needed he simply came forward and helped as long as there was necessity for him, then when the task was finished he would, just as silently, fall back on his usual chores.

But inside the house he came nearer showing interest. At fifteen he was as good at all kinds of housework as his mother, even to cooking. During the times when she was ill he carried on her work so well that her absence was scarcely noticed, except that the meals were sometimes late. Joe could never accomplish any kind of work rapidly. He puttered through his boyhood and puttered at everything which he undertook. It was the slowness which arises from slowness of wits, his hands and feet were active and skillful enough, once his slow-conceiving mind functioned.

He evinced interest in but one thing, aside from his mother, and that was in reading. His interest in it was repressed but genuine. His mother and the cowboys had taught him to read and since his mind was not crowded with any other interests or studies he learned rapidly. Even in boyhood he read all the newspapers and the few magazines which found their way to the ranch. The only trips he took by himself were horseback rides to a neighboring ranch, eight miles away, to borrow a book. And he asked for each one in a hesitating, half frightened way.

"Futile!" Big Bill would snort. "Never be able to take care of himself. Always will be puttering around somebody, and somebody always will have to look after him. Both of 'em. Him and her. Futile!"

But the years were bringing many changes to the old Indian Territory, as Joe grew up. Oklahoma had been carved out of the western part of it and was now thickly settled. Then the "Big Pasture" finally was opened to homestead entry. Thousands of people flocked in, almost over night.

The ranches disappeared; they had always used government and Indian lands, and now these were taken from them. Big Bill Barde, one of the last to be routed, started moving his outfit to the Texas Panhandle. He offered to take Joe and his mother with him, as soon as he got the new ranch under-way, but before he could come back for them he died suddenly of pneumonia. His heirs knew nothing of Joe and his mother, and besides they were not inclined to carry any "dead timber."

So Joe and his mother, perforce, began a life of drifting about the country, from place to place and from state to state, wherever they could find employment—for the two of them. They always went together. If the mother found work it was part of the bargain that Joe also should be taken on, and work for "his keep." It is doubtful if either of them ever received more than a few dollars in cash during the twenty years that followed. The mother would get a job cooking for some farmer or threshing crew, Joe would do chores, and for their joint work they would receive their food, some sort of place to sleep, what rough clothes they urgently needed, and perhaps a little credit at some store.

Joe could never ask for a job; his mother had to find work for him. Yet he worked well at anything he was given to do. "He would almost make a good hand if he wasn't so dadblamed slow," the farmers all said. "He can do most anything you set him at, but he takes all day about it."

But the passing years were leaving their mark on Joe's mother. She seemed to change character under the repeated blows of her harsh and unsatisfying existence. Her illnesses were becoming more frequent and the storms which flashed in her eyes were far less repressed. Occasionally the storms now broke through her restraint; furiously when they first came on, only to be succeeded within few minutes by helpless weeping. Like Joe, though few had guessed it for years, she was, as Big Bill had expressed it, "futile."

But the storms broke more often, and her sullenness cropped through. People who did not understand her began to fear her; they whispered that she was going insane. She learned of the whispers. And the wild outbreak which resulted caused the family for which she and Joe were then working to call the authorities and have her committed to the state hospital for the insane.

Joe was dazed. He scarcely comprehended. It took his slow moving mind several days to fully understand. He knew only that he was being separated from his mother, and was bereft and helpless.

A few days later the county judge who had committed his mother felt a hesitant pull at his sleeve, just as he started into his chambers. He turned to face Joe—his face trembling more than usual, his eyes haggard.

"I want to be sent to the same place you sent my mother," Joe managed to say in his frightened, futile way. The judge stared, as mingled comprehension and sympathy came to him slowly. "Do you mean to say that you want to be sent to the insane asylum?" he asked. There was a trace of admiration in his voice.

"Yes," said Joe. "I want to be near her." The judge summoned a judicial air. "Well, I guess we can accommodate you. You are not insane, exactly, but I guess any doctor would admit that, mentally, you are not all there."

So Joe came to this hospital, where his mother was confined. He could not be in the same building with her, nor see her often. They were both patients, legally committed, and rules are rules. Even when permitted to visit her in her ward he could see her only in the presence of attendants and not for long. But he could hear of her, could know that she was fed and sheltered in comfort, that she had clean clothing to wear and very light work, for the first time in all the years that Joe could remember. It comforted him.

But it tore his heart that he could not take her "home" as she so often begged, although they had no place in the world to go even if she had been released.

As for himself, Joe did not seem to care. He could not be released, either, but he had never known a home, and would not have missed it if he had one, for he had never felt an interest in anything in all his life, except his mother and his reading.

The hospital authorities put Joe to making up the dormitory beds, and sweeping and cleaning. He still puttered, but no woman could have done more tidy work. The other men on the ward would have their share of the work completed while Joe was still painstakingly in the midst of his, but his beds and floors would shame the maids in a good hotel.

Joe was still a woman in inclinations; a trembling-faced, frightened woman in spite of his sex. And all of his futile time he brooded about his mother; so near and yet so separated from him. When he was with her for a brief visit there was no outward show of affection; no kisses, no hand-clasps, no endearing words. But she would have one of her storms after he had been led away, and his face would tremble more than ever for a day or two.

Now Joe's mother is going to die; the mother for whom his love was so great that he followed her even into the sombre, life-long immolation of the insane asylum, with but one pitiful comfort possible—that of being near her. And Joe is dazed; she is all that he has, all that he has ever had. Even his beloved reading can not interest him. If sympathizing fellow-patients offer him a paper or a magazine he starts up as though frightened, only half comprehending, his face trembling; and a fumbling hand pushes the offering away.

Joe's mother has been moved into one of the hospital wards. Joe is taken in to see her every day. But she is very ill. She recognizes him with her eyes only, or not at all.

In his futile way Joe realizes that whatever of interest and affection he has in life will go out with her; that most of him will die when her life-tortured spirit tears itself free.

A part of him, the physical part, will live on; making beds in the hospital dormitory, cleaning and polishing floors, while the slow years drag into other years. But whatever of human interest he may now possess, whatever of good there may be in him, will be under a mound in the hospital cemetery.

Joe's mother is dead. An attendant got the news over the telephone and shouted down the corridor, "Joe, your mother is dead." He did not intend to be heartless. That is the way it is always done.

Joe gave a little choked cry, stumbled into his room and shut the door. He did not go down to dinner. He stayed in his little room with the door closed.

This afternoon he stumbled into my room. "I—I don't want her buried here," he said haltingly. "It isn't fit for the likes of her. She—she was a good mother. We've got a lot in a cem'tery somewheres. She told me once. But I can't remember. Her family's buried there. I don't know who they are but I want her buried with them."

He shifted his feet and swallowed convulsively, his face twitching more than ever. "If I only had some money, or if—if the boys could make it up. I could pay 'em back sometime. I don't want her buried out there in a pauper's grave. It isn't fit for the likes of her. She was a good mother."

I could not help him; none of the patients can help him. You can not make up a burial purse in an insane asylum ward.

Joe is trying hard to think. Face and hands tremble with the effort. "I'm going to write," he says. "Maybe I can find out. I'm going to write." He stumbles back to his room. He is still in there. He will not write. There is no one to whom he can appeal. We are sorry for Joe. But what can we do?

I know just what will happen. Joe's mother will be taken to the hospital morgue and kept for a day or two while hospital authorities make a futile attempt to locate relatives. Then her body will be buried decently in the hospital cemetery, and Joe will not be told. He will not know; it is better for him not to know. He will not worry long about where she is buried. He will soon forget all questions regarding that. He will remember but one thing; that his mother is dead. He will go on making beds in the dormitory, puttering around, futile.

A new squaller, just arrived and locked in a room near Joe's, is thrusting his head through the little square opening in his door and bawling out his opinions of the attendants, the patients and the world in general. But Joe does not hear him. Joe is thinking of his mother.

Futile. Futile.

CHAPTER XVII

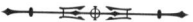

JAM ON THE BRAKES

I COUNT the months over, like the telling of beads. Six months here, yesterday. Six more months to go. Then—where?

Wait. Pull up short. Eradicate that groove which the sly feet of Old John Barleycorn have tramped into your brain, then start counting the months, and asking "Where?"

Easy, Man. You are here for a definite purpose; forever to erase from your being every trace of that mad, overwhelming, periodic, mental craving for liquor, whatever the cost. Better another year, two years, than to go back to that.

Let restlessness and the bitter gall of life, as you are compelled to live it, drive you out just a short month too soon and all that you have paid for emancipation will be irrevocably lost. And that price is such that, once paid over, it can not be called back. The stigma of legal insanity clings; it is ineradicable. Your surrender of position, of friends, of wide acquaintance, of a certain standing among men will have been worse than useless. You will go out, tainted, to begin life over, at middle age, under new surroundings, unknown, and stamped as further convicted of weakness, to add to the other taints.

Steady there! Steady. Steady. Hold fast.

The ward physician is helping me. Together we are trying an experiment in the redemption of a rum-seeped soul, the rehabilitation of a dipsomaniac. We hope it will result in scientific information to the medical world which will bring about the redemption of that class of almost uniformly brilliant men and women who develop the mental craving.

Steady, plodding men and women almost never become periodics. It is those with tingling nerves, highly sensitive and relentlessly driving, who become dipsomaniacs.

Even among the alcoholics here, few are typical periodics.

It was the wise old physician in charge of the first "liquor-cure" hospital at which I was ever a patient who tried to tell me what was necessary for my permanent rehabilitation. I had taken the full thirty day course of treatments, at $75 a week, and was ready to start for home, when he called me into his office.

I felt fully cured. My head was clear, my blood bounding, I had gained weight, I felt no scintilla of desire for alcohol. I was convinced that I was clean of the habit.

But the physician faced me with a serious expression. "Mr. ——— we have cured you of your physical craving for alcohol," he said impressively. "But I have studied your case closely. While as yet you do not realize it you are in the early stages of a periodic craving. In a short period of time we can not cure that; no one in the world can cure that through medical treatment. And you have all the characteristics of one of the most typical periodics I ever encountered, although I have treated thousands of alcoholic cases. I want you to know the truth. Put yourself where it will be impossible for you to secure liquor for six months or a year, and I believe you can win."

My egotism pranced right up on its hind legs. What was he playing me for—a sucker? Was he trying to frighten me into staying there, at $75 a week, for six months or a year? I had too much sense for that. Catch me failing for so obvious a trick. That was out. I was clean; clean.

I brusquely refused. I thought him a grafter. Now I know he was a scientist. But what a price I have paid for that information.

The ward physician here and myself are putting that suggestion into practical operation. But we are adding a safety indicator to it. I will be kept confined here until both the physician and myself are convinced that the mental groove is erased.

Then we will test our convictions. Into my room will be brought a bottle of whiskey. It will be left there, I will have free access to it. I can see it, smell it, taste it if I wish, and thus test out whether it has any further power to call me.

And the test will be conducted at a time when normally I should be suffering from my periodical craving. Yes those craving paroxysms occur at regular intervals, three weeks apart, and lasting for several days. They are not weakly, namby-pamby things for scoffers to laugh at. If not assuaged with liquor they become spells of physical and mental illness. My mouth drools saliva, my stomach and intestines seem cramped, and I become bilious, nauseated, and in a shaky, nervous funk.

I have not yet conquered those periods. A whiff of whiskey breath, a month ago, proved that. A visitor came down the hallway past the open door of my room, on his way to visit another patient. His breath reeked. It swirled through my open door and slapped me in the face. I went wild. That whiff put me in bed, nervously ill. No I have not erased that brain groove, as yet.

But the attacks are far lighter than when I was committed. Sleepless nights and a highly nervous state for two or three days are the remaining symptoms when no smell of liquor is around. I believe that in six months more I can smell liquor, even taste it—and leave it alone.

Then the outside world, a squaring of the shoulders, cauterization of any sensitiveness to suspicions and rebuffs, a supreme call on manhood—and what?

Common Sense and the members of my family agree on the answer. "Grab your typewriter," they say. "Hustle straight for a cabin in the woods, beside some lake or stream. Hide your trail from crowds and bootleggers."

"Indulge your love of fishing and outdoor life. Let your typewriter earn the meals you cook and eat. Beat back along safe and sure lines. Don't strain your moral fiber beyond its strength."

Common Sense and my family are in perfect accord. But that cadaverous pest, Better Self, always bobs up with, "What about Constance?"

And my ambition, somewhat emaciated, slyly jogs my elbow. "What about going back into your own world and licking it? Have you guts? Or are you a yellow quitter?"

I shoo the pestiferous and disturbing bunch out the room and turn to my typewriter. Its clacking exorcises the troublesome trio for a few minutes, until I remember with a start that it was Constance who made a trip from my home city to bring me my typewriter, and who persuaded the superintendent to risk disturbing discipline by having such an unaccustomed machine on the ward.

Then the three come trooping back, and I flee to the exercising porch to escape them. They vanish when I mingle with the other denizens of the ward. They refuse to mingle with the insane.

As I pass down the hall the latest Squaller has his head thrust through the square opening in the door of his room, and is shouting his opinion of the hospital in a throaty, raucous voice.

"What kind of a dump is this, anyhow? I been in three hospitals before this and they were all better'n this. This is the worst of the lot. What kind of a place are you running here? Treating me this way. If I could get at you I'd fix you. You just remember that, you blistering loonies. (Time out, for a string of profanities.) Think I'm crazy? Think I'm going to stay here? (Time out for a string of obscenities.) I got a long memory. I'll remember it. I'm going to get out and fix you. (Time out for a string of all known kinds of invective.)

He sees me standing listening in awed silence, and he turns the vials of his wrath on me.

I go right away from there.

As I pass the open door of the bath room a new patient is being examined and "tabbed." "They told me they was taking me to visit an old friend, and the first thing I know I am being locked up here," he is explaining to the attendant. He is taking it with chuckling good humor. In the words of the older patients there does not seem to be much the matter with him.

I reach the porch and sit down beside Nelson, the irrepressible, and Mundy, one of the parole men. The hot, stifling summer weather has brought a veritable invasion of swift, little, black bugs which the patients call "oat bugs." They have overrun the hospital like the Huns overran Europe.

"Doggone it," says Nelson. "I never saw the like. Why last night, in bed, they was so thick that a line of 'em would form under one side of my back and all heave at once, like fellers raising the timbers of a bridge, and darned if they wouldn't heave me right out of bed. Yes sir. Heaved me out nine times. But I managed to crawl back every time and they finally got discouraged." He chuckles at his own wit.

Mundy gets up and walks around him, examining him critically. "You don't seem much scarred up from all that bumping," he hazards.

"No sir," Nelson retorts, grinning. "You see there was so many of 'em on the floor that they made me a nice, soft cushion to light on. I killed thousands of them but their friends was all so busy picking up the remains that I always had a soft spot to light on." The listeners applaud.

Nelson is congratulating himself on getting sent here at just the proper time. He admits that he was making and selling liquor at home, before he got "the tremens."

A few days after his arrival here federal operatives swooped down on his home county and made a mighty haul of stills and their owners. "If I'd a been there I'd a probably been among those present," he says. "And me so blame crazy with liquor that I'd a probably told them birds the truth."

But now two hotly arguing patients are demanding my services as referee in a learned dispute. Since I am permitted the dignity of using a typewriter they conclude that I must know a great deal. "Say, this nut claims that Pike's Peak is in Missouri," says the little wizened one. "I know it's in Kansas 'cause you drive to it right out of Omaha. Tell him it's in Kansas."

"It ain't," retorts the fish-eyed one. "It's in them Missouri hills, right out from St. Louie; ain't it?"

I know the penalty of being a referee here, but I am in a reckless mood and take a chance. "You are both wrong. It's in Colorado, and you drive to it out of Colorado Springs."

The wizened one looks at me in disgust. "You're a fool," he snorts, and stalks off. Fish-eye casts a baleful glare at me. "You're crazy as a bedbug,"

JAM ON THE BRAKES

153

he sneers, and stalks off. Tiddle-de-dum. A prophet is never without honor save among his own people.

I escape to my room to do a little writing before the call of bedtime. I am not allowed to do any writing after that. But I manage to "bootleg" considerable reading after the lights in my room are turned off and I am supposed to be in bed.

There is a hall light just outside the door of my room and by sitting near the doorway but far enough back to be out of sight of the night attendant I can read at night, if the print is large enough.

When the attendant starts down the hallway I can hear his shoes on the concrete floor and I skitter into bed and hide my book or magazine beneath the sheet.

I have never had to put it to the test but I believe the attendant would suffer a case of voluntary temporary blindness if he should catch me in the act. You see he enjoys reading and I keep him well supplied with the magazines which Constance sends me.

Constance. Darn it; her name is always bobbing up.

CHAPTER XVIII

Debts of Others

THEY are taking Carol to the Hydro today and the other patients on the ward are already coming out of the sulks and beginning to feel happier. Many of us will sleep better tonight, and all of us will feel far less irritable when we no longer can hear or be kept jumpy by Carol's horrible caterwauling.

For Carol has "gone cat."

Not only does be believe he is a cat; so far as any part of his consciousness is concerned he is a cat, and he is desperately fighting a cat's natural enemies in a cat's way, with a cat's squalls and yowls, and at times with a cat's rasping scream of death-pain.

For several days Carol has been locked in a side room which was designed and built for the purpose of keeping the screams of "squallers" from reaching the ears of other patients and ruffling their nervous condition. Even the little, square opening in the door, through which the attendants can peer before entering the room, is covered with heavy plate glass, half an inch thick and protected by steel wire webbing. But Carol's piercing voice penetrates even the thick walls of this room and jars the nerves and disturbs the sleep of patients as far away as the dormitory.

All last night, from dusk to daylight, Carol, as a cat, fought a pack of savage dogs for his life. This morning he evidently has escaped from his deadly peril. He has been emitting mews that bear a note of contentment. At times he even purrs, but his mews, purrs and pfist-pfist have a penetrating quality which is almost as bad as his cries of cat combat.

He "went cat" three days ago. In the intervening seventy-two hours there has not been a space of five minutes when he was not uttering feline noises. The men's nervous control, always precarious, is tottering.

"He don't belong on this ward. He ain't fit to stay here," Collins says, nervously petulant. "They ought to keep him in the Hydro all the time or send him to one of the noisy wards. That's where he belongs."

Collins is not sympathetic with cats. His own obsession has nothing to do with cats. When he has a disturbed spell his delusion is that he must carry out some supreme sacrifice in order to make his peace with God. So he is impatient with Carol's cat psychosis.

This morning the ward physician came and looked through the glass into the room where Carol was eating his breakfast. Carol was crouched on all fours in the middle of his bed, his face thrust down into his plate, eating his food just as a cat would, and emitting the spitting growls with which a belligerent tomcat warns away any possible poachers from his food.

The physician's face was grimly sympathetic. Carol has always been a likable boy before these hallucinations began riding him; quite rational, courteous, and apologetic whenever he felt that he was at fault in any way. His mind has been clouded at times but the cat obsession had not found its way into his brain. Then suddenly he became a cat.

"Send him to the Hydro," the doctor ordered, almost gruffly. Then he came into my room with a weary air.

"You are writing something about sterilization, aren't you?" he asked. "Well there is a first class object lesson for you. Sins of the fathers, and a damned clear case. We have known this was coming. He was condemned to it when he was conceived—the spirochete in his ancestry, and he is paying a part of the bill his ancestors should have paid. Just write that down for the public to read."

I understood. He is one physician who bitterly condemns the sterilization law, as written, in spite of the fact that he is unequivocably in that group which believes the vast majority of insanity cases are due to heredity.

"From his immediate parents?" I asked.

The doctor threw up his hands with a gesture of helplessness. "How can I tell? Probably his father, but it might have been his grandfather on one side or the other. Not a chance in the world for that boy to get out and have children, and yet some fools would sterilize him while his father and mother and sister and brother are still outside and productive. The chumps would dump off all civilization's responsibilities on that helpless product of other people's follies, and feel that by sterilizing him they had straightened out the whole sorry mess." He scowled angrily and tramped out.

Yes, Doctor. I have written it down for the public to read, just as you said it. And I am restraining an almost irresistible impulse to enlarge on and praise a part of it and lash viciously at that part with which I do not agree. I am restrained only by the fact that the public will pay close attention to what you say, because you are not only a physician but one who has had long experience in studying and treating the insane. But the same public would attach little if any credence to what I might say, because I have been declared insane; and hence it is possible that at any time I might lose my rationality and have a disturbed spell.

"You never can tell about such fellows. You know he was sent to the asylum, once." Can't I just hear people saying that?

Neither am I going to comment on the case of Collins who is obsessed with the idea that he must make some supreme sacrifice in order to placate God. I merely set out the facts as they appear.

Collins has not been here very long. He was brought in very weak from the loss of blood. He had been attending a "protracted revival meeting" in a country community, conducted by a revivalist who continually wrought up and inflamed the emotions of his hearers.

Collins had become fired more and more with religious fanaticism as the meeting continued. One night the evangelist preached from the text, "If thy right hand offend thee cut it off and put it from thee."

That quotation may not be quite correct. It has been many years since last I read the passage, and no Bibles are permitted on the wards of this asylum. Religious reading and discussions lead to bitter disputes and even fights among the majority of patients, and almost invariably rouse the religious maniacs to dangerous frenzies, the officials say.

To the untrained mind of Collins that command to "cut it off and put it from thee," was to be taken literally. The preacher had said so; had pounded the point home with intemperate and inflammatory zeal. Collins returned to his home, procured a butcher knife, went out into his night-darkened yard, prayed—and attempted to desexualize himself.

He fainted from pain and loss of blood before he succeeded. But his family could not convince him that he was wrong. He was madly determined to complete the mutilation at the first opportunity. To his inflamed mind his sex impulses were a fleshly offense to God. He forgot that the God he believes in must have endowed him with those impulses. The preacher's words still rang in his ears. So he was committed here. He arrived on a stretcher.

He is now recovered. He goes about quietly most of the time. He has learned that he must do that. But we feel that he is watching and waiting for an opportunity to carry out some act of supreme sacrifice to placate the God which his disturbed mind pictures to him.

We watch Collins. We do not relish the possibility that one of us may be the central figure in some sacrifice that he may believe he hears God ordering him to make.

And you never can tell about such fellows. You know he was sent to the insane asylum . . . .

Wait, . . . back up, . . . just what am I saying?

Am I just? Am I broad? Am I fair? Or am I bitter at the way the public judges me, yet guilty of meting out the same judgment to others?

Oh, but my case is different . . . . But isn't that the frantic cry of nine patients out of ten in every hospital for the insane?

And I had planned to go back to my home city and lick it into accepting me. I slump limply back in my chair. I can not write any more. That sudden collision with a realization of where I stand in the eyes of others has smacked the fight out of me, hauled me up short, snatched a fatuous dream away from me and left me gasping and groping.

An attendant passes the open door of my room. He looks at me keenly. "What's the matter? Are you sick?" he asks, sharply. I pull myself together and stumble to my feet. "No," I answer. "Just thinking."

"That's the trouble with a lot of you guys. You think too much," the attendant retorts succinctly. He goes on down the hallway, glancing keenly in at each door. He has to watch us all; you see we are all patients in a hospital for the insane.

He is a new attendant. He does not know me very well yet. But does he? Am I competent to judge?

God! ". . . to see ourselves as others see us!"

They are taking Carol to the Hydro. He is tightly swathed in sheets from crown to soles to keep him from biting, or clawing with hands or feet. He is having one of his paroxysms. We know what he will do when he is in a paroxysm, and so we do not fear him.

Collins passes my door, quietly, unobtrusively. He is not in a paroxysm. He is apparently thinking deeply. So I watch him—narrowly.

The attendant passes back past my open door. I am standing still, thinking. So he watches me—narrowly.

Chapter XIX

Dress Parade

Tomorrow is a national holiday and the ward has been seething with activity all day, preparing for it. For on holidays the hospital goes on dress parade.

Bath day, shave day and hair-cutting day were all merged into one, this morning. Attendants shouted orders; spurring the patients to quicker and more vigorous action; whooping things up like a mate on an old time river steamboat, with a big loading confronting him.

Rooms, halls, dormitory and day room were given an extra furbishing. Tomorrow morning "best clothes" will be issued to all patients who expect visitors and to all others who will be taken to the park for the "celebration."

And the visitors will be here. On every holiday they come. There will be trembling faced old mothers, visiting their vacant minded or delusion-ridden sons, and bringing fruits, cakes or candies. God bless them.

There will be wives coming with a new shirt, tie or socks for husbands, long here—and here for long God bless them

And there will be the baldly curious, sight-seeing visitors, offensively peering, and hunting for those delightful shivers.

God . . . (choke—splutter)—bless them. (Confound it. The rules prohibit profanity.)

The advance guard of this type of mental vandals came through the ward a few minutes ago; just after everybody had been shaven, shorn and made presentable for company. They went away looking disappointed. Nobody, not even an epileptic, had a fit while they were here. And most of the patients looked almost human. Then everything was so spick and span.

Even Whizbang Mabel and her co-cursers were unaccountably silent. But one voice disturbed the air.

A withered, little old lady in the ward across the court was singing. She was seated at her window, facing the sunshine. Her quavering voice came haltingly, as though her memory was yearning backward into past years as she sang

"Darling I am growing old; Silver threads among the gold, . . ."

I am sure they went away disappointed.

But they will have one thing over which they can clack their tongues and smack their lips. Some of them were from the university in my home city, and they recognized me. They did not know that I am here. But they know it now. They recognized me with little surprised—and anticipatory—cries. One of them, a woman, ran the skewer in me and twisted it around in the wound. She came right into my room."

Aren't you Mr. ——? Why I did not know you were here. I've read so much of your lovely work. Do they let you write here? Well isn't that nice?" And how she will spread the news at home! Guurhh!

Tonight, though, we of the best ward, or rather the best of us on the best ward, have been having a real treat. We, the favored ones, were permitted to sit up long past bedtime. We have been listening to a blow-by-blow account of a fight in which, strangely, neither patients nor attendants were participants.

In fact the fighters wore gloves, so it couldn't have been much of a fight although it was ballyhooed as being for the championship of the world. We are not accustomed to that sort of fight. Here the fighters never wear gloves.

But how the men did enjoy that broadcast. They gathered in a ring, five deep, around the radio stand, and rooted for their individual favorite, even as you and I. One fellow was standing off by himself, in a sort of exalted daze, and fighting both sides of that distant prize fight. He would execute every blow, just as the broadcaster announced it.

By the end of each round he was as exhausted as either of the fighters could have been. But he would come up gamely for the next round. Right, left, counter, block, duck and clinch. Finally he knocked himself down, stayed down till the count of nine, got up and raised his own hand in token of victory.

Now that is what might be called actively enjoying a prize fight.

I must sneakingly confess that my own muscles were surreptitiously flexing as I "helped out" my own favorite. And at countless radios, throughout the nation, the John Joneses, Bill Smiths and Tom Whites were flexing their muscles and mentally helping out their favorites, and came out of it perspiring and tired. However that patient was superior to the rest of us. He had a double track mind. He was standing in the shoes and fighting the fight of both the fellows who were cuffing away in that distant ring. And he did not have 75,000 frenzied spectators to help him.

A good time was had by all.

But the night attendant hustled us into bed immediately after the prize fight ended. He did not want any reenactments of the bout, with two excited patients impersonating the principals.

Betting was high on the ward before the broadcast began. The patients backed their favorites to the limit. "I betcha a thousand dollars Stribling whips him," ferociously shouts Wild Bill, the former prize fighter. "I betcha a thousand he won't," retorts Mathews who was a lumberjack by profession"

I betcha ten thousand he will," screams Bill, smacking his fists together. "I betcha twenty thousand he won't," shrieks Mathews.

"You fellahs are both crazy," cuts in a cynic. "This fight is all in the bag. Of course they've got it all framed up. They always do."

Where have I heard that before? I am sure it was not in an insane asylum.

But some of the bets were more substantial. I know of at least ten boxes of safety matches which changed hands on the result. Safety matches are legal—or rather illegal—tender here. The rules prohibit any of us having matches of any kind. The attendants are permitted to carry safety matches, which can not be ignited by striking them against anything except the prepared side of a match box. The rule probably saves much bedding and some undertaking services.

But, like some other things the possession of which is prohibited, safety matches are bootlegged. The attendants know it. On this ward they manage to forget it if the patient who gets the safety matches is "safe." But on many of the other wards, they have to be more careful.

A patient who has a pipe or cigarette and no match is supposed to go to the attendant for a light. The patients who manage to secure matches are very careful not to give any to patients who can not be relied on. Some one might fire his bed and the rule against having matches would be strictly enforced for a time—and the bootlegger might be caught.

The prospect of hearing the fight broadcast put the patients in a high, good humor all evening. Shafts of characteristic wit scintillated frequently.

It was Nelson, the irrepressible ex-bootlegger, who started it. We were sitting on the exercising porch after supper when he suddenly drawled "I wonder what Herbert Hoover would say if he knew I was here." There was a whoop and the wits joyously piled to the assault. "I know what he'd do. He'd just remember yore record in France and say, Just send him some beans and barbwire and he'll feel right at home,'" one fellow giggles. Nelson spent three daredevil years "over there."

"You won't dare let him know you are here, Nelson," another wit jibes.

"He might let your wife know where you are and you would be in a worse fix than you are now."

"Shucks, you fellows act like Nelson didn't have but one wife. He's been about some," says another.

So the badinage went tossed hither and yon, until the attendant sent to bed those patients who were not permitted to stay up for the fight news.

One of the most enthusiastic fight fans of the ward, Young Roberts, did not get the fight news tonight. But he was too wildly happy to care about that. He was in an automobile, speeding toward his distant home; released today after six years here. And his father and mother came for him. They have been loyal all those years. And I believe he is the kind well worth being loyal to.

He came here a high school boy. I am not sure what toppled his mental balance. "Too much study," the patients say, and they add that he was wildly demented for months after his arrival. His mind cleared very slowly, but apparently surely.

He came of an excellent family; intelligent, broadminded, refined and courteous. He is one of the handsomest young men I have ever seen. Yet, he is thoroughly masculine, a man's man, highly popular with the other patients as well as with the hospital authorities.

He is a star athlete. He played on the hospital baseball team, which is composed mostly of attendants. And that team has mopped up about every other amateur team within automobile radius. Attendants are a mighty athletic set of young men, as a rule. They have to be.

For the long months that I have been here Roberts has appeared to be fully, sane in every way; not only sane, but keenly intelligent. He was almost invaluable on the ward. In addition he is a talented musician and has several expensive instruments, supplied by his parents.

Of course he has been longing to go home. But the physicians wanted to be sure of his permanent recovery. They kept him here under observation for a long period.

For some time he has sensed that he would be sent home soon, although no one would tell him so. The attendants and physicians are the best sphinxes in the world when a patient wants to know when he is going home. It is a good rule, although few of the patients think so. The officials do not want to raise hopes too high. A patient may he getting along so well that the authorities are planning to send him home, then at the last minute have another disturbed spell or develop symptoms which make it necessary to keep him for further observation.

Roberts had no idea that he was to go home today. He was at work in the art department when the superintendent 'phoned him that his parents were waiting for him. He was wildly happy and rushed to the ward to get his belongings. But even at that he took time to make a full round of the ward, shaking hands with the men and wishing every one good luck.

Nelson received a different sort of surprise today. He had hoped to be paroled home within a few days. Today the physicians discovered evidence that the spirochete is at work in his system. He may have to stay here for a course of treatments. "Three months more, at least," he told me despondently. "Three more months in Hell." Nelson has spent much time in army and civilian prisons. He grinningly admits that he is "stir broke."

"But this place isn't stir," he says. "It's plumb ' Hell. If I get snakes again I'm just agoing to choose the good old county jail for mine. Me for this place never again."

But it takes even more than the prospect of few more months in here to cure him of his irrepressible nonsense.

He says that if he has to stay he will use the time in organizing the alcoholics here into the Hospital Booze Bugs, an organization to promote "better and more realistic vaudeville."

"We'll just put these old booze hounds on the stage and let them sing 'Sweet Adeline,' an, 'Show Me The Way To Go Home.' Can't anybody sing them two better or more naturally than they can. Why there ain't one of them that hasn't sung them songs a thousand times."

He has plenty of material from which to select his members. The number of alcoholics here continues to grow steadily.

There are grades of society even on the receiving ward. But birth, social training, former standing and refinement have nothing whatever to do with the circle to which a patient finds himself inexorably assigned.

In the relentless grading of the insane hospital you find yourself judged by "how much you have the matter with you." Soon you are associating most of the time, with those who have about as "much the matter" with them as you have.

Once I saw pecans being graded by being thrown upon a vibrated screen, or rather a series of screens, one beneath the other. The top screen had wide slits in it. Each of the lower screens had successively narrower slits. As the screens were shaken the very largest nuts remained on the top screen, the smaller ones dropping through the slits. As the shaking continued the smaller nuts kept dropping toward the bottom, each screen retaining those which were too large to pass through its slits.

The nuts here are graded in the same way. They are just shaken by their fellow patients until they drop down to their own rationality level.

Many of them are no more conscious of being shaken down to their own stratum than were the nuts in the pecan plant.

The elite stratum here is composed of the better fellows who are "under cover from the law," the men who have recovered and are about to be paroled home, and the more intelligent alcoholics who have safely weathered the delirium stages.

Ahem, and a couple of preenful poses. That puts me in the very tip top of society here.

The qualifications for acceptance in this haughty group are ability to take or pass a joke with unfailing good humor—at least without undue resentment; sufficient intelligence to play bridge, chess or checkers without introducing rules of your own or carrying away fisticuffs-producing grudges; rationality enough to discuss the daily news without telling the other fellow he is a fool or crazy as a loon; and tolerance with the frailties of others sufficient to entitle you to be known as a general good fellow. I wonder how many men on the outside could fully qualify.

It pays to be in the upper crust. Most of its members have rooms of their own, are permitted to attend the ball games, film shows and dances, and are tacitly permitted to carry matches, keep a little change in their pockets and even have watches.

I carry my own watch. Constance brought it on one of her visits. She had one of her stormy spells, that day, when I refused to decide definitely what I intend to do when I go out. She wept angrily and long, flung vixenish accusations at me, and finally flounced away from the hospital with her eyes red and sulky, but she left my watch and a supply of typewriter paper.

That combination of recriminative storminess, angry weeping—and kindness, helped so much, and is still helping, to give me an unpeaceful mind.

CHAPTER XX

Hung on the Line

THE dress parade was a huge success. All the spectators are agreed on that. They say the patients were so beautifully handled and so surprisingly well behaved.

Even most of the patients agree that the picnic at the park was a treat. The food was both good and plentiful. Of course there were some disadvantages. The patients were seated well apart on the grass, each one had a separate paper plate, and there was little opportunity to grab tempting morsels from the other fellow. That took some of the zest out of the unusual dainties. In addition attendants were everywhere and even good, soul-satisfying bickerings over the food were suppressed.

But the potato salad, pickles, cakes, iced lemonade and ice cream cones partially recompensed for the good behavior that you were forced to maintain. All of these were delightfully unfamiliar.

No knives or forks were supplied with the paper plates of food. Each patient was given a spoon, but these were carefully collected later. Even the handle of a spoon may be sharpened to a dangerous edge if rubbed vigorously on a concrete walk for a sufficient length of time. The authorities do not believe in tempting any suicidal or homicidal patients beyond their strength.

Every patient on every ward who was not actually sick or too feeble or violent to go was taken to the park. There were about fifteen hundred patients and two hundred attendants and employees present. And such a decking out of the patients as had taken place on each ward before attendants marched them down to the park, where spectators could see! It is for dress parades and the coming of visitors that the state provides a good supply of "best clothes" on every ward.

Of course some of the patients felt a little uncomfortable in their unaccustomed best clothes. One big fellow felt quite abused about it. "This here's the first time I been allowed to get on the dirt in six months," he complained. "And I can't even lay down in it. Me, I like plenty of good old dirt. If you want to be healthy just get plenty of dirt in your pores. That's natural, ain't it? Look how long people used to live. They got plenty of good old dirt in their pores."

Members of the upper crust are disdainful of such a view. Some of them actually objected to the dust which the wheels of the spectators' automobiles stirred up. As if spectators should be expected to miss any of the show they had come to see, just because some of the patients had on newly laundered shirts, sent them from home.

There was plenty of entertainment at the picnic. It opened with the singing of America, led by the hospital orchestra. Old Man Jeffries refused to remove his hat while the song was being sung. One of the other patients remonstrated with him. "Say, that song's not for the likes of us," Jeffries retorted. "If this is the land of the noble free I'd like to see a place where folks are kept cooped up."

There was square dancing for the better patients, egg, sack and hobble races, a fat men's race, a fat women's race, and a tug of war. Whizbang Mabel was the individual athletic star of the day. She won the fat women's race, going away, but it was in a special event that she won her proudest acclaim. There was an individual tug of war between herself and a man opponent. But Whizbang squared her Amazonian shoulders and dragged that man across the finish line like dragging a catfish out of the creek. And the man weighed but little less than she does.

She was pridefully puffed up for the rest of the afternoon and at night when the usual chorus from the women's ward across the court opened its concert Mabel's mighty bellow was absent.

She was satisfied with the amount of attention which she had attracted during the day.

Her place was partially filled by the man on Ward 3 who is always dying. He has been "dying" almost every night for weeks. He did not get to go to the park, so he died with unusual vigor during the early hours of the night.

"Oh-ooo, I am dying!" he would boom. "Can't you do something for me? Oh-ooo, I am dying."

Finally one of the patients on this ward, whose room is just above that of the man who is constantly dying, pressed his face against the bars of the window and howled back. "Well hurry up and die, you noisy nut, and see if we care."

The "dier" has not accepted the invitation. Aside from a paralyzed left side, a crippled right hand and a twisted brain he seems to be in good condition.

In spite of the large number of patients gathered for the festivities in the park there was but one determined break for freedom. That was by a woman. I had a ringside seat for that feature.

The women were seated in one part of the park and the men in another, with a roadway between them. This road was the deadline between the two sexes and was patrolled by attendants. For some reason, or for divers reasons, the patients, both men and women, seemed to congregate along the sides of that roadway.

I don't know how I came to be right at the men's edge of the road, unless it was because I am a little nearsighted.

Suddenly a woman sprang from among the other women patients and dashed straight down that road. For the moment there was not an attendant in front of her.

Then I saw another woman patient dash into the roadway and launch herself in a flying tackle at the knees of the fleeing woman. She landed with all the precision of a Notre Dame half back stopping an Army ball carrier, and the result was similar except that she clung on longer. Two attendants had hold of the would-be escaper before she released her hold.

After seeing Whizbang Mabel pull that man across the tug of war line, and after watching that flying tackle I am in favor of granting women full equality. If we don't they will come and take it anyway.

That was but one of the jolts which pet convictions of mine received during the day.

I had previously believed that every man and woman who is locked in is wild to get outside, even if for but a short time. Two of the men on this ward, who are in good health, had to be forced to go to the park. "No sir. I don't want to go to the park. I'm not agoing," one of the men said. "What's the use to get out for just a little while if they aren't agoing to let me go home. They've kept me locked up for the last six months now. When I go out again I wanta go home."

The other man made every possible excuse to avoid going. One of the attendants, an observing fellow, preached me a little homily on that. "He is just afraid to go. Some of these fellows are afraid of anything to which they are not accustomed. That fellow was terrified for three months after he got in here, but now he has become accustomed to life on the ward and is not afraid of it any longer. But he is afraid to go out because he does not know just what might happen. Some of them are like that on most of the wards."

Then that attendant heartlessly stepped on the corns of the most cherished conviction that I have formed here. "A few of these patients who grieve the hardest because they are not permitted to go home wouldn't go if they had the chance." I gulped, and blinked.

"They are nearly all old people, though," he continued. "They have become settled here and are afraid of any change.

"Why in one hospital where I worked there was a nice, old man. He was sane but just in his dotage. They kept him in the parole ward. He had been there for several years. He had lost all track of his relatives, but he was always grieving because he could not go home.

"But he had a son in Pittsburgh who had been trying to locate the old man. Finally he traced him to the hospital and after communicating with the superintendent, came to get him.

"The son was fairly prosperous; had a good home and no family except a wife and one daughter. He was prepared to give the old man every comfort. He never suspected that the father would object to going, but he certainly did. And he had been begging for three years to be sent home. But he changed his mind when his chance came. He said he had become so used to the hospital that he could not be satisfied anywhere else. It took his son three days to overcome his objections and persuade him to leave.

"I never could make up my mind whether it was because the old man did not want to feel dependent on his son, whether he was afraid to face the wife and daughter, or whether he was afraid of just any change of any kind. I believe it was the latter."

I am inclined to agree with him. I know of a case where three old women wept piteously at being removed from the county poor farm, where they had been living several years, and taken to a far more comfortable and attractive home for aged women. Somehow they felt that their lives were being pulled up by the roots.

I know that my own dear old mother declines to live with any of her children, although they are abundantly able and willing to care for her, and she is growing feeble.

She says she wants a home of her own, "where she feels free to do whatever she wants to do." Perhaps some of the aged, even in this hospital for the insane, if they came face to face with impending removal, might discover that their lives are somewhat rooted here.

I know that some of them are waiting, just waiting, to get the dreary business of living over with.

There is Old Man Noyes. He is stone deaf. No earthly sound ever reaches him. He lives in a world all his own. How it is peopled I do not know. No one knows, except Noyes. But not one of us believes that it is peopled with anything in the nature of a hallucination or an obsession. He is very old. His body is badly bent with years. Yet he is full of kindly, thoughtful little acts, that indicate that he is gentle and lovable.

He sits in his room all day long. His eyes are fixed on something far away. What it is we do not know. He may be dreaming of loved ones now gone out of his life. He may be visioning whatever there may be beyond the grave. He never tells us. He speaks very seldom and then in the uncertain, hesitating tones of one who has not been able to hear his own voice in many years.

He is shut in with his thoughts. He can not have one confidant. So he dreams on, his eyes always on something far away.

And outside his room mills the heterogeneous life of the ward. There is Nelson, the ex-moonshiner and bootlegger and ex-husband of several women. We can guess the kind. Nelson was not apt to be particular. There is Boxx, hard muscled and hard jawed mechanic, who started life as an orphan newsboy, and graduated into apprentice mechanic, enlisted navy man, marine engineer's assistant, aviation mechanic and owner of an automobile repair shop by the time he was twenty-six. Yet he is an unbending and uncompromising Christian.

It is his solemn boast that he never touched liquor. He deplores profanity and is scathingly abhorrent of anything which savors of immorality, even a pert, risque joke.

There is Corry, a six foot, handsome alcoholic who has done all of the things which Boxx hates, and does not abhor or regret a one of them, even his addiction. His parents had him committed in an attempt to save him, but he frankly does not intend to be saved. His Lights o' Love are strung all the way from Manhattan to Galveston beach. He has written to one of them to hire an attorney and try to get him released. I do not know what kind of promises he made her. He had the letter smuggled out, he tells me.

There is Sunderland, one of the finest men imaginable when his mind is not under a cloud. We all love him then. Just now the cloud is drifting its tortuous way across his mind. In a few days he will have to be taken to the Hydro. We are sad at his affliction, but avoid him. In his disturbed spells his delusion is that he has been unkind to, critical of, or harsh toward every one he knows, and he is pitifully repentant of it. He will corner the other patients and plead with them to forgive his figmentary offenses. He will write remorseful letters to the physicians, begging them to forgive and forget any critical thing he has said about them. He has never yet said one unkind or critical thing about the physicians, or anyone else. Charity itself could not be kinder in its judgments of others. But his tortured mind tells him that he has; and how bitterly he suffers!

His periods of normality last for several months or a year. In one of these he was discharged from a hospital in another state, came to this state, opened a decorating shop and was building up a thriving business when the cloud returned. He was committed here.

When he is not disturbed he is one of the most valuable men on the ward. He is intrusted with the bathing of all new patients and knows how to handle them diplomatically. He can often quiet a mildly raving patient and he is always the first one to rush in and restrain one in a paroxysm of violence. Now the other patients must soothe him and try to relieve him of his delusional remorse.

Within a day or two Sunderland will have to be taken to the Hydro. He will probably stay there several months before he becomes fully rational again. He fell to the floor three times today, completely unconscious. That shows that his paroxysm has nearly reached its peak. We will miss Sunderland.

Then there is ———, but why catalogue their characteristics and their frailties? Why hang their portraits on the wall and baldly label them for all to see? Their prototypes, except that their characteristics are less exposed to view, more retiring at the insistence of reason, more hidden at the demands of exigency, are walking the streets of every city, sit in every luncheon club, greet friends in every chamber of commerce and slap the backs of pals in every trades union.

There is but one portrait that I have a right to hang on the line. It is my own, and I can not paint that, with truthfulness and accuracy. I can not limn the lines which mental habits have engraved on my own character. I do not know myself.

Wanted: a portrait painter.

But do I want one?

CHAPTER XXI

The Spin of the Wheel

AGAIN I am counting the slow months over, as they drop reluctantly from the calendar of the year.

Nine months here. How many to go?

But this time I am doing it with better justification, with far better warrant for hope. It won't be long now. Just a few more months; and the months are slipping by a little less hesitantly, and with far less of racking perturbation of mind.

Nature, abetted by a set-jawed determination on my part, is gradually eliminating that scar in my brain which Alcohol tramped into it. The obsessionary recurrent periods of craving have become anemic, rather feeble things; able to jar me but little, nervously, and scarcely at all physically.

Nine long months out of Booze's grasp. Yo ho! and a bottle of grape juice. The heat of summer is far behind. The frosts of fall are here. I may not be "out of the trenches by Christmas," but some time soon after the New Year offers a clean page on which to begin imprinting the history of my second life. I believe, and the ward physician believes, that it will be safe to put my physical and mental rehabilitation to the test; to place in my room a bottle of whiskey where I can see it, think about it, smell it and taste it, to learn if its power over me has been wiped out.

The physician has assured me that as soon as he is convinced that the obsessionary periodic craving is gone beyond recrudescence, the locks will click behind me, as I go out to reshape my life.

Whoops for that. Loud whoops, and several of them, in spite of the fact that as yet I can not know certainly whether I will measure up to the full stature of a man, or whether I must remain longer on the receiving ward.

But I do know this; I have settled that question of which way I shall take. I have routed the grinning gibbons which jibed me with the question, "Which way out?" I have grappled with them and tossed them out onto their collective ears.

I have seized that pestering pair, Common Sense and Better Self, knocked their two heads together, boxed their ears soundly, and kicked them flying after their fellow nuisances.

I summoned the courage to do this through the simple expedient of coming to a determined decision. A determined decision will rout most vexatious problems.

I know where I am going when I "go home." I have blue-printed the plans for the first floor of my second-life structure, which I must build from the basement up. I have sealed those plans with a vow that nothing can swerve me from the course which they lay out for me.

I was not put to the necessity of getting rid of Ambition—that drooping fellow who was always jogging my elbow and asking, "What about going back to your own world and licking it into accepting you?

When I had kicked out the others and turned to settle with Ambition I found that he was already dead. Those carrion carriers, the thrill-seeking visitors, had killed him. He could not survive their avid licking of their lips when they found me here, nor the knowledge that they scarce could wait to scuttle back home before starting their tongues to clacking.

But it was a young, new attendant here who really gave Ambition his final blow, although the poor fellow's condition was very low before that. The attendant is a member of a family with which I was well acquainted before I was sent here. His mother is the best single handed gossip spreader in my home city.

He was not at all surprised to see me. He addressed me by my familiar given name but never offered to shake hands. His manner was exactly that of the average man toward an insane patient. And his brother had been one of my luncheon club associates back home.

I put a question to him, grimly. "Did you know that I was here?"

"Sure," he answered tartly. "Everybody knows it. What did you expect?" He turned away so as not to be bothered with me longer. He did not want to be compelled to listen to any of the troubles of a "nut."

Ambition passed away, right there.

No, I am not going back to my world and try the impossible task of licking it into accepting me.

I decline to be ostracized. And I refuse to be Oslerized. So I have decided to be Horace Greeleyized.

I am going west, for my second start in life. High up in the heavily timbered mountains of New Mexico, sixty miles from the nearest town and twenty miles from the nearest highway, is a well built, comfortable, three-room cabin. A mountain stream, fed from the snows above and hiding many a speckled trout, runs brawling by it. A narrow road, passable to a capably-handled automobile, winds through miles of timber to reach it.

It belongs to a friend of mine. He has tendered me the use of it for a year. When I wrote him, hesitantly, and asked him if he would lease it to me for that period he replied with an offer of its free use so effusively that I was unkind enough to suspect that he believes I will trouble him less when I am two thousand miles from him than if I should go back to my home city. Fie on me! He bought the place for a summer fishing camp, but his wife declined to visit it. She likes her vacations in fashionable summer hotels.

When I go home I will take only time enough to recover legal use of my car. I will pack it with just such things as I will need in a mountain cabin, sixty miles from a barber shop—or a bootlegger—and fifteen from the nearest neighbor. There will be one exception; my typewriter shall have the place of honor beside me on the front seat.

Thank the Fates, my love of fishing and hunting has preserved to me a fair measure of woodcraft and familiarity with camp life.

And when I turn my car westward from my home city the man that I was, as the kind of man that I was, will cease to exist. To all intents and purposes he expired when I was checked in on the receiving ward. His history ended there. And the tempo of the song of busy affairs was not jarred out of measure by a single beat, when he dropped out. How we all do overvalue ourselves.

When I reach the cabin I will sink my ax into the nearest dead pine and cut plenty of fire wood. I will carry water from the brawling stream, build a fire in the little iron stove in the kitchen and prepare plenty of hot water. I will scrub the pine floors and walls of the three rooms. With boiling water I will rout the little, red ants which always gather in such a long-deserted cabin. I will open the doors and windows and let sun and mountain air do their good work

I will wash the enameled plates and platters and bowls, scour the kitchen utensils, wash the windows and even trim the wicks in the kerosene lamps. I will try to make everything spick and span.

Then I will send for Constance. She says she will come. I will meet her at the railway station, out where the white desert and the foothills meet.

In the little town we will buy clean linens and bedding and some simple drapes for the windows, and bacon and flour and canned goods and the other necessities for camp life.

Then we will hunt up some benign old minister in the little town. We will be married, quietly, quite matter-of-factly. And we will drive sixty miles into the mountains, to a three room pine cabin, fifteen miles from a neighbor and three hundred from a night club.

She has never lived anywhere except in teeming cities. She never saw a mountain cabin and has seen the mountains only from the window of a Pullman car.

And we will learn if the stern crucible of that mountain cabin life can fuse two as gratingly different characters as ours; melt the whole, skim off the sorry dross of the lives we both have been living, and somehow, miraculously, bring about a regeneration and a unity which might endure.

We will learn if she can be content away from the tawdry glitter of city "party" life, away from beauty parlors and permanent waves, silk pajamas and corn whiskey cocktails, and jazz dance music and good shows. (At the expense of some flirtatious old man.)

We will learn if she is willing to get up in the morning and help cook breakfast for two, instead of staying in bed until early afternoon, then languidly 'phoning the restaurant in the next block to send up grapefruit and dry toast and coffee, to which she can add a "spike" of liquor, left over from last night's party.

We will learn whether she can be happy taking a bath from a foot tub on a pine floor instead of from a porcelain bathtub on a tiled floor—with plenty of bath salts and the temperature of room and water graduated to a nicety.

We will learn if she can be satisfied with continual association with just one man, and without association with the over-colored and chattering women of her usual group.

And we will learn if I am broad and adaptable enough to sympathetically bear with and soothe her periods of stormy weeping; diplomatic and self-controlled enough to remain silent and apparently contrite through her tantrums of tongue-lashings and recriminations, and man enough to forget her lack of fineness of mental fiber, remembering only her splendid loyalty and constancy in the hours of my desperate need.

We will learn whether I can smile and be attentive to her chatter when she interrupts me right in the middle of the formation of some ear-pleasing phrase in the story I am writing, in the hopes that I may persuade some publisher to buy it, and thus give me the money to continue our experiment in double regeneration.

We will learn if two people, middle-aged, and moulded hard into characteristics which inevitably clash, can remould themselves at the unaided call of that world-old attraction between members of the opposite sexes which in our youth we called love.

If the miracle can be accomplished then within a year or two our address may be, Mr. and Mrs. ———, Some Quiet Home, Comfortable City, U.S.A.

If the call of the old life becomes too strong for her, if the strain of forced association with just one man becomes more than she can stand, if she decides to go back to the beauty shops, the comfortable bathrooms, the nighttime carousal hours and the daytime sleeping and dawdling hours, and to the men and cocktails of her past life, I will take her to the little desert town, put her in the Pullman car and kiss her a final goodbye. I will not go back to the life to which she is returning. I can not do that. If I so much as hung around its borders for six months I probably would be ready to go back to the asylum—for a lifetime stay. And all that I have undergone would be for nothing—worse than nothing for there would be the stigma of an added fall.

After the train has disappeared into the white desert, taking her back to the glitter of the old life, I shall go back to the little mountain cabin, until I have completed the regeneration of myself.

In the meantime the mills of the law, turning lackadaisically in some distant city, will grind out an unnoticed divorce. We have agreed that if either of us goes back to the old life the other will not contest a divorce action. For if natural attraction and our desire for each other can not remould us, certainly the flimsy bonds of the law could not.

Then the building of a new life will be greatly simplified for me. The pallor of the hospital ward will have been replaced by the healthy brown of outdoor life. That troublesome interim in my history can be shied around easily. I have just been "in the mountains, free-lance writing, for a year or two." Even a conscience more squeamish than mine could find justification for such an evasion, under the circumstances.

Nine months on the receiving ward. A few more months to go. Then our experiment in dual regeneration.

Place your bets, Ladies and Gentlemen. Fate, the croupier, inscrutable and detached, as all good croupiers should be, is about to spin the wheel.

Which will come up? A home for remoulded personalities, fused into contended union; or a party woman under the bright lights and a fellow trying to pound out his regeneration on the keys of a typewriter, by the light of a kerosene lamp in a mountain cabin?

Or will it be a woman who has tried to aid a man in his remaking and seen him falter, swerve, and go back to the receiving ward?

I can not tell. Constance can not tell.

Place your bets, Ladies and Gentlemen. Fate, the croupier, is about to spin the wheel.

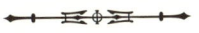

Afterword

William W. Savage, Jr. and James H. Lazalier

MARLE WOODSON, deemed cured of drink, left Eastern Oklahoma Hospital early in 1933. He traveled to New York, wearing whiskers and under an assumed name, to be feted by his publisher. On March 9 he appeared in Tulsa before the same judge who had committed him in 1931 and had his rights restored. Thereafter, he devoted himself to establishing a library for the inmates at Eastern. He had observed that they had little to occupy their time, and he noted the dearth of any sort of reading material. Soliciting discards from the collections of his friends, he traveled often between Tulsa and Vinita, bringing boxes of books and magazines for the hospital.

Sometimes during the summer of 1933, Woodson inadvertently slammed a car door on his arm, and when the wound gave no sign of healing, doctors discovered advanced bone cancer. It spread quickly from arm to shoulder to lungs. By September, his friends knew he was dying. As he wrote to one of them at mid-month, "I cannot give you any idea as to how long it will take me to end my little job of living. . . . For the time being it is all very painful and weakening and monotonous." Nevertheless, he was capable of sending "a cheery greeting."[1]

Marle Woodson spent his final days at Eastern Oklahoma Hospital. He died on the morning of October 5, 1933. Funeral services were held on October 7 at the Methodist church in Vinita, and Woodson was buried at Fairview Cemetery. Pallbearers were members of the Vinita Lions Club. Survivors included his mother and a younger brother, living in Dallas, and a sister, living in Oklahoma City.[2]

Was Constance at the service, or at the graveside, faithful still? We cannot know.[3]

Eastern Oklahoma Hospital, like the others in the state system, continued to be overcrowded and understaffed through the thirties. Nearly half of the inmates who left the facility still did so as passengers on the Gray Wagon. Survivors still fretted over the sterilization law, which, in 1933 was amended by the Oklahoma legislature to apply to prison inmates as well as mental patients, as reformers continued to try to eliminate undesirable behaviors through eugenics.[4] A half century later, no one was prepared to say with any degree of certainty how many Oklahomans had been sterilized according to the law's provisions, but estimates ran into the hundreds. And a half century later, no one pointed back to the 1933 law to compare Oklahoma reform under populist governor William H. "Alfalfa Bill" Murray with race-thinking in Hitler's Germany. The state legislature repealed the sterilization law in 1983.[5]

Behind the Door of Delusion spent time on the reading lists for some college sociology courses; but eventually the public's memory of it faded, as did the name of Marle Woodson. Owing to a post–*The Grapes of Wrath* reaction against any recollection of the 1930s, Oklahomans have taken pains since World War II to eradicate as much of the cultural history of the Depression era as they can; and for that reason Woodson must stand with such Oklahoma writers as George Milburn, Jim Thompson, and William Cunningham, all waiting to be rediscovered by the people of whom, and for whom, they wrote. Each dealt, in his own way, with the dispossessed and the alienated, the victims who had no place to go.[6] The dispossessed and the alienated are as much with us in the 1990s as they were in the 1930s, so it would seem appropriate to give new voice to Marle Woodson and his contemporaries. If, as he wrote, Fate is the croupier, we must all acknowledge our status as bettors.

Notes

1. Quoted in Mary Hays Marable and Elaine Boylan, *A Handbook of Oklahoma Writers* (Norman: University of Oklahoma Press, 1939), p. 214.

2. "'The Door of Delusion' Is Closed for Marle Woodson." *Tulsa Tribune*, October 6, 1933, pp. 1,6. Brief notices appeared in *Tulsa World*, October 6 and 8, 1933.

3. Said an anonymous writer about Constance in "Miscellaneous Brief Reviews," *The New York Times Book Review* (September 25, 1932), p. 12, "The reader can accept her as real or imaginary, as he likes, but he will probably guess that if she were a real person the author would not have written so intimately about her. And if he accepts her as real she is likely to make him feel dubious about 'Inmate's' future."

4. "Oklahoma Puts Sterilization Law Into Effect," *The Literary Digest* (May 12, 1934), p. 17.

5. *Laws Thirty-Ninth Legislature, First Regular Session—1983*, Chapter 71, p. 216. Murray paroled more than 2,000 convicts on the condition that they leave Oklahoma. The same could not be done with hospital inmates.

6. Milburn, Cunningham, and Thompson were novelists and short-story writers, but the same could be said of Oklahoma poets like John Berryman and Welborn Hope. See Frank Parman, "Sons of Bankers," in Parman (ed.), *Aggregate Images: An Assemblage of Poems, Art and Reviews* (Norman: Cottonwood Arts Foundation, 1989), pp. 3–4. Milburn, Thompson, Berryman, Hope, and journalist-turned-novelist Edward Anderson shared Woodson's taste for alcohol, and a couple of them wrote novels reflecting their views on the problem. See John Berryman, *Recovery* (New York: Farrar, Straus and Giroux, 1973). Jim Thompson, as Oklahoma director of the Federal Writers' Project, responding in 1939 to a question about *Behind the Door of Delusion* from national FWP director Henry G. Alsberg, said, "State residents, and competent book reviewers, . . . doubt many of the statements and the value of the book as a piece of literary work." Alsberg to Thompson, June 16, 1939, Oklahoma Historical Society Archives, WPA Writers Collection, Box 1. Nevertheless, editors Angie Debo and John Oskison left a reference to the book in the first edition of the WPA's *Oklahoma: A Guide to the Sooner State* (Norman: University of Oklahoma Press, 1941), p. 222, and it was still there when a revised edition appeared in 1957, by which time Thompson had published his novel, *The Alcoholics* (New York: Lion, 1953), a burlesque involving doings at a California sanitarium named El Healtho.